A COURSEBOOK

ON

SCIENTIFIC AND
PROFESSIONAL WRITING

IN

SPEECH-LANGUAGE PATHOLOGY

Second Edition

Singular Textbook Series
Series Editor: M. N. Hegde, Ph.D.

*Articulation and Phonological Disorders:
A Book of Exercise, Second Edition*
by Ken M. Bleile, Ph.D.

*Clinical Methods and Practicum in
Speech-Language Pathology*
by M. N. Hegde, PH.D.

*Applied Phonetics: The Sounds of American
English, Second Edition*
by Harold T. Edwards, Ph.D.

*Applied Phonetics Workbook: A Systematic
Approach to Phonetic Transcription,
Second Edition*
by Harold T. Edwards, Ph.D., and
Alvin L. Gregg, Ph.D.

Instructor's Manual for Applied Phonetics
by Harold T. Edwards, Ph.D.

*Introduction to Sound: Acoustics for
the Hearing and Speech Sciences,
Second Edition*
Charles E. Speaks, Ph.D.

*Speech-Language Pathology: Assessment
Resource Manual*
by Kenneth G. Shipley, Ph.D., and
Julie G. McAfee, M.A.

*Introduction to Communication Sciences
and Disorders*
Edited by Fred D. Minifie, Ph.D.

*Anatomy and Physiology for Speech
and Language*
by J. Anthony Seikel, Ph.D., Douglas W.
King, Ph.D., and David G. Drumright, B.S.

*Clinical Speech and Voice Measurement:
Laboratory Exercises*
by Robert F. Orlikoff, Ph.D. and
Ronald J. Baken, Ph.D.

Language and Deafness, Second Edition
by Peter V. Paul, Ph.D., and
Stephen P. Quigley, Ph.D.

*Study Guide for Language and Deafness,
Second Edition*
by Peter V. Paul, Ph.D.

*Instructor's Manual for Language and
Deafness, Second Edition*
by Peter V. Paul, Ph.D.

Diagnosis in Speech-Language Pathology
Edited by J. Bruce Tomblin, Ph.D.,
Hughlett L. Morris, PH.D., and
D. C. Spriestersbach, Ph.D.

Neuroscience of Communication
by Douglas B. Webster, Ph.D.

*Introduction to Clinical Research in
Communication Disorders*
by Mary H. Pannbacker, Ph.D., and
Grace F. Middleton, Ed.D.

Optimizing Theories and Experiments
by Randall R. Robey, Ph.D., and
Martin C. Schultz, Ph.D.

*Professional Issues in Speech-Language
Pathology and Audiology*
Edited by Rosemary Lubinski, Ed.D., and
Carol Frattali, Ph.D.

Clinical Methods and Practicum in Audiology
by Ben R. Kelly, Ph.D., Deborah Davis,
M.S., and M. N. Hedge, Ph.D.

A COURSEBOOK

ON

SCIENTIFIC AND PROFESSIONAL WRITING

IN

SPEECH-LANGUAGE PATHOLOGY

Second Edition

M. N. Hegde, Ph.D.

California State University-Fresno

SINGULAR

★

™

THOMSON LEARNING

Africa • Australia • Canada • Denmark • Japan • Mexico • New Zealand • Philippines
Puerto Rico • Singapore • Spain • United Kingdom • United States

NOTICE TO THE READER

COPYRIGHT © 1998 Delmar. Singular Publishing Group is an imprint of Delmar, a division of Thomson Learning. Thomson Learning™ is a trademark used herein under license.

Printed in the United States of America
4 5 6 7 8 XXX 03 02 01 00

For more information, contact Singular Publishing Group, 401 West "A" Street, Suite 325 San Diego, CA 92101-7904; or find us on the World Wide Web at http://www.singpub.com

Library of Congress Cataloging-in-Publication Data

Hegde, M. N. (Mahabalagiri N.), 1941-
     A coursebook on scientific and professional writing in speech-
language pathology / M.N. Hegde. — 2nd ed.
          p.   cm. — (Singular textbook series)
     Includes bibliographical references
     ISBN 1-56593-868-2 (spiral bound)
     1. Speech disorders—Authorship—Handbooks, manuals, etc.
2. Language disorders—Authorship—Handbooks, manuals, etc.
3. Medical writing—Handbooks, manuals, etc. I. Title. II. Title:
Scientific and professional writing in speech-language pathology.
III. Series.
     [DNLM: 1. Writing. 2. Speech-Language Pathology—education. WZ
345 H462s 1997]
RC423.H3829   1997
808'.06661—DC21   97-23984
                                          CIP

Contents

Preface to the First Edition   x
Preface to the Second Edition   xi
Introduction   1

**PART A. FOUNDATIONS OF SCIENTIFIC
AND PROFESSIONAL WRITING**   **5**

A.1.   BASIC RULES OF USAGE   **6**
A.1.1.   Do Not Turn a Plural Into a Possessive   6
A.1.2.   Do Not Turn a Possessive Into a Plural   6
A.1.3.   Use the Correct Forms of Possessive Nouns   8
A.1.4.   Use the Possessive Forms of Pronouns Correctly   14
A.1.5.   Distinguish Contractions From Possessives   14
A.1.6.   Use Unusual Singulars and Plurals Correctly   16
A.1.7.   Use a Serial Comma   20
A.1.8.   Do Not Use a Serial Comma When You Write Only Two Parallel
          Terms and Connect Them With a Conjunction   20
A.1.9.   Use a Comma to Separate Parenthetic Expressions When You Do Not
          Use Parentheses   22
A.1.10.   Place a Comma Before a Conjunction Introducing an Independent
          Clause   22
A.1.11.   Join Independent Clauses With a Semicolon When the Clauses Are
          Not Joined by a Conjunction   24
A.1.12.   Use a Dash to Set Off an Abrupt Break or Interruption   24
A.1.13.   Agreement   26
A.1.14.   Use Modifiers Correctly   34
A.1.15.   Do Not Use Pronouns Whose Referents Are Not Clear   36
A.1.16.   Do Not Break a Sentence Into Two   36
A.1.17.   Do Not Turn an Adjective into a Noun   38
A.1.18.   Do Not Turn a Noun into a Verb   38
A.1.19.   Use the Proper Case of Pronoun   40
A.1.20.   Make Sure a Participial Phrase at the Beginning of a Sentence
          Refers to the Grammatical Subject   40

A.2.   BASIC RULES OF COMPOSITION   **42**
A.2.1.   Design a Broad Outline of Your Paper   42
A.2.2.   Design Headings and Subheadings of Your Paper   44
A.2.3.   Write Paragraphs That Express Related Ideas   46
A.2.4.   Do Not Write Paragraphs That Are Too Long   48

A.2.5.   Do Not Write One-sentence Paragraphs   50
A.2.6.   Begin and End Most Paragraphs With Transitory Sentences   52
A.2.7.   Use the Active Voice   54
A.2.8.   Prefer the Shorter to the Longer Sentence Structures   54
A.2.9.   Use Positive Terms   56
A.2.10. Avoid Too Many Qualifications   56
A.2.11. Use Definite, Specific, and Concrete Language   58
A.2.12. Eliminate or Replace Unnecessary Phrases   60
A.2.13. Avoid Redundant Phrases   68
A.2.14. Avoid Wordiness   74
A.2.15. Keep Related Words Together   76
A.2.16. Maintain Parallelism   78
A.2.17. Avoid Dangling Phrases   80
A.2.18. Avoid Shifts Within and Between Sentences   82
A.2.19. Make Quotations Count   84
A.2.20. Do Not Overuse Quotations   86
A.2.21. Do Not Include Islands of Quotations   88
A.2.22. Do Not Begin a Sentence With a Quotation   88
A.2.23. Use Quotation and Punctuation Marks Correctly   90
A.2.24. Do Not Overuse Quotation Marks   90
A.2.25. Give References for All Direct Quotations   92
A.2.26. Reproduce Quotations Exactly   94
A.2.27. Integrate Quotations of Less Than 40 Words With the Text   94
A.2.28. *Block* Quotations When They Have 40 or More Words   94
A.2.29. Show Correctly the Changes in Quotations   98
A.2.30. Use Latin Abbreviations Only in Parenthetical Constructions   100
A.2.31. Avoid Euphemism   102
A.2.32. Avoid Jargon   102
A.2.33. Use the Terms Ending With -ology and (and Some With -ics) Correctly 104
A.2.34. Avoid Clichés   106
A.2.35. Avoid Colloquial or Informal Expressions   106

A.3.   COMMONLY MISUSED WORDS AND PHRASES   108
A.3.1.   Affect and Effect   108
A.3.2.   Alternate and Alternative   108
A.3.3.   Allusion and Illusion   110
A.3.4.   And/Or   110
A.3.5.   Farther and Further   110
A.3.6.   Incidence and Prevalence   112
A.3.7.   Inter- and Intra-   112
A.3.8.   Latter and Later   114
A.3.9.   Secondly and Thirdly   114
A.3.10. Since and Because   114
A.3.11. Elicit and Evoke   116
A.3.12. Elicit and Illicit   116
A.3.13. Compare to and Compare with   118
A.3.14. Compare and Contrast   118
A.3.15. Effect and Impact   120
A.3.16. Focus and Analysis (Study)   120

A.3.17. There and Their 122
A.3.18. Accept and Except 122
A.3.19. Baseline and Baserate 124
A.3.20. Proof and Support 124

PART B. SCIENTIFIC WRITING **127**

B.1. PRINCIPLES OF SCIENTIFIC WRITING **128**

B.2. WRITING WITHOUT BIAS **131**
B.2.1. Write Without Gender Bias 132
B.2.2. Write Without Prejudicial Reference to Disabilities 133

B.3. FORMAT OF SCIENTIFIC WRITING **136**
B.3.1. Give Correct Margins 136
B.3.2. Use Appropriate Line Spacing 137
B.3.3. Use Acceptable Computer Printers and Typefaces 137
B.3.4. Do Not Overuse Boldface 138
B.3.5. Use the Recommended Type Size 138
B.3.6. Use Acceptable Paper 138
B.3.7. Type Correctly the Title Page of a Paper for Publication 140
B.3.8. Type Correctly the Title Page of a Class (Term) Paper 141
B.3.9. Type the Page Header and the Running Head Correctly 142
B.3.10. Write an Abstract on the Second Page 143
B.3.11. Begin the Text on Page Three 144
B.3.12. Number the Pages Correctly 145
B.3.13. Reprint the Corrected Pages 145
B.3.14. Use Correct Indentation 145
B.3.15. Give Correct Space or No Space After Punctuation 146
B.3.16. Use the Headings Within the Text Consistently 147
B.3.17. Write Out Abbreviations the First Time You Use the Term and Enclose the Abbreviations in Parentheses 154
B.3.18. Do Not Start a Sentence With a Lowercase Abbreviation 154
B.3.19. Do Not Write Out Units of Measurement When a Number is Specified 156
B.3.20. Write Out Units of Measurement When a Number is Not Specified 156
B.3.21. Add the Lower Case Plural Morpheme *s* to Plural Abbreviations Without an Apostrophe 156
B.3.22. With Abbreviations, Use the Period Correctly 158
B.3.23. Use Roman Numerals Only When It Is an Established Practice 158
B.3.24. Use Arabic Numerals for All Numbers 10 and Above 158
B.3.25. Use Numerals for All Numbers Below 10 in Specified Contexts 160
B.3.26. Write Out in Words Numbers Below 10 Under Specified Contexts 162
B.3.27. Write Out in Words Any Number That Begins a Sentence 164
B.3.28. Combine Words And Numerals in Specified Contexts 164
B.3.29. Distinguish Between a Reference List and a Bibliography 166
B.3.30. Cite the Author's Last Name and Year of Publication in the Text 166
B.3.31. Cite Both Names in the Text When a Work Has Two Authors 166
B.3.32. Cite Works With Three to Five Authors Using All the Authors' Names Only the First Time 168

B.3.33. Cite Works of Six or More Authors by Only the First Author   168
B.3.34. Distinguish Works of Multiple Authors Published in the Same Year   170
B.3.35. Join Multiple Names With *and* or &   172
B.3.36. Cite Multiple Authors With the Same Last Name With Their Initials
         Every Time They Are Cited   172
B.3.37. Cite Multiple Works of the Same Author in a Temporally
         Ascending Order   174
B.3.38. Attach Alphabetical Suffixes to the Same Author's Multiple
         Publications in the Same Year   174
B.3.39. Within Parentheses, Arrange the Last Names of Multiple Authors
         in Alphabetical Order   176
B.3.40. Begin the Reference List on a New Page With a Centered,
         Uppercase, and Lowercase Heading   178
B.3.41. In the Reference List, Arrange References in Alphabetical Order   180
B.3.42. Arrange Multiple Works of the Same Single Author From the
         Earliest to the Latest Year   180
B.3.43. Alphabetize the Titles of Several Works of the Same Author
         Published in the Same Year   182
B.3.44. Alphabetize the Different Authors With the Same Last Name
         According to Their Initials   182
B.3.45. Indent the First Line of Each Reference Entry by Five to Seven
         Spaces and Type the Second and Subsequent Lines Flush Left   184
B.3.46. Use the Specified Abbreviations in Reference Lists   184
B.3.47. Journal Articles in Reference Lists   186
B.3.48. Books in Reference Lists   188
B.3.49. Edited Books and Chapters in Edited Books in Reference Lists   190
B.3.50. Reports from Organizations and Government Agencies in
         Reference Lists   190
B.3.51. Proceedings of Conferences and Conventions in Reference Lists   192
B.3.52. Convention Presentations in Reference Lists   192
B.3.53. Unpublished Articles, Theses, or Dissertations in Reference Lists 192
B.3.54. Cite the Electronic Sources Correctly   194
B.3.55. Cite Correctly an Individual Work With an FTP (File Transfer
         Protocol)   195
B.3.56. Cite Correctly an Individual Work on Telnet   195
B.3.57. Cite Correctly a Journal Article in a Database   196
B.3.58. Cite Correctly a Part of a Work From an Electronic Source   197
B.3.59. Cite Correctly an Entire Journal in a Database   197
B.3.60. Cite Correctly an Entire Thesis or Dissertation in a Database   198

B.4.   **FORMATS OF RESEARCH PAPERS**   **200**
B.4.1.   Parts of a Research Paper   200
B.4.2.   Write the *Review*, the *Methods*, and the *Results* of a Completed
         Study in the Past Tense   206
B.4.3.   Write the *Discussion* Section of a Completed Study in the
         Present Tense   206
B.4.4.   Write the *Review* Section of a Research Proposal in the Past Tense 206
B.4.5.   Write the *Methods* and *Expected Results* Sections of a Research
         Proposal in the Future Tense   208

PART C. PROFESSIONAL WRITING   211

INTRODUCTION TO PROFESSIONAL WRITING   212

C.1.   DIAGNOSTIC REPORTS   213
C.1.1.   An Outline of a Typical Diagnostic Report on a *Child Client*   214
C.1.2.   An Outline of a Typical Diagnostic Report on an *Adult Client*   216
C.1.3.   Anatomy of an Assessment Report   218
C.1.4.   Sample Diagnostic Reports   225
C.1.5.   Practice in Clinical Report Writing   245
C.1.6.   Reports Written as Letters to a Referring Professional   303
C.1.7.   Practice in Writing Reports as Letters   311

C.2.   TREATMENT PLANS   317
C.2.1.   Comprehensive Treatment Plans   318
C.2.2.   Brief Treatment Plans   322
C.2.3.   Individualized Educational Programs   331

C.3.   PRACTICE IN WRITING TREATMENT PLANS   337
C.3.1.   Comprehensive Treatment Plans   348
C.3.2.   Brief Treatment Plans   346

C.4.   PROGRESS REPORTS   363
C.4.1.   Progress Reports Written as Letters   375

C.5.   PRACTICE IN WRITING PROGRESS REPORTS   379
C.5.1.   Progress Report: *Written as a Letter*   404

C.6.   PROFESSIONAL CORRESPONDENCE   407
C.6.1.   A *Thank You* Letter   408
C.6.2.   A *Referral* Letter   409

C.7.   PRACTICE IN WRITING PROFESSIONAL CORRESPONDENCE 411
C.7.1.   A *Thank You* Letter   412
C.7.2.   A *Referral* Letter   416

BIBLIOGRAPHY   417

GLOSSARY   419

Preface to the First Edition

Teaching and learning to write in a technical and professional language is an important part of education in speech-language pathology. However, students often do not begin to acquire acceptable writing skills until they enroll in clinical practicum or in graduate research seminars in which professional and scientific writing are required. But many students are not adequately prepared for such writing.

Students who have taken courses on writing offered in other departments still do not have adequate technical and professional writing skills. To write well, students need to write and receive specific feedback. Students should rewrite and have multiple opportunities to practice the same type of skills and receive feedback every step of the way.

There are many books on writing, but few that give opportunities to practice writing as the examples are given. Most instructors know that simply asking students to read various books on good writing does not generate writing skills. Also, most writing courses are designed to teach rules of grammar, not writing. However, a good writer need not recite rules of grammar. Therefore, I have designed this new type of book which I call a *coursebook*. I have used this book in teaching technical and professional writing skills to undergraduate students with good results. This book makes it possible not only to show and tell what acceptable writing is but also to have students practice such writing immediately, on the ^cing pages of the same book.

I hope that instructors of courses on writing, assessment and diagnosis, ^duate seminars on research methods, and clinical supervisors will find this ^ helpful in teaching technical and professional writing skills to students. In *ntroduction*, I have described the different methods of using this book. I ^me comments and suggestions from students and instructors who use this

Preface to the Second Edition

In 1994, it was my hope in writing this new type of coursebook on professional and scientific writing that instructors and student clinicians would find it useful in teaching and learning writing skills in the classroom itself. The response of instructors around the country has been overwhelmingly positive. Many instructors have commented that there has been a need for this kind of book and that the coursebook method is more effective in teaching writing skills than are traditional books on writing.

A significant change in the second edition is that it reflects the scientific writing style of the fourth edition of the *Publication Manual of the American Psychological Association*. Several new rules of usage and their correct and incorrect exemplars have been included in this second edition. In many cases, the number of exemplars have been increased to give students more opportunities to practice appropriate writing skills. Additional examples of problematic writing sampled from students' writings have been included. Professional writing exemplars, including assessment, treatment, and progress reports, have been streamlined. A glossary of clinical terms used in report writing has been added to facilitate students' correct usage of those terms. The design of the book has been improved to make it more functional for students.

I thank my colleague Dr. Celeste Roseberry-McKibbin who has given me many suggestions for improving the book. As instructors of a course on scientific and professional writing offered in the Department of Communicative Sciences and Disorders at California State University-Fresno, Dr. Roseberry-McKibbin and I have received many suggestions from our students to improve the book. I am thankful to all those students. I am thankful also to Jenny Carter—an exceptional graduate student who taught the course on scientific and professional writing—and in the process, helped me revise the book for this second edition.

I am grateful to the editorial and production staff at Singular Publishing for their extraordinary support and hard work on completing this second edition in a timely manner. My special thanks to Angie Singh, Marie Linvill, Sandy Doyle, and Lynnette Hunter.

INTRODUCTION

WHAT IS A COURSEBOOK?

A *coursebook* is a new type of book. It is a book that students not only read, but write on as well. It includes features of a textbook, a book of exercises, a resource manual, a laboratory manual, and an instructor's manual or handbook. By combining elements of different types of teaching tools, a coursebook becomes a unique and practical teaching tool.

The most important aspect of this coursebook is the way the left-hand and right-hand pages are designed. Most left-hand pages show specific examples of general, scientific, or professional writing. In many cases, both the incorrect and correct versions are shown. The corresponding right-hand pages require the student to write correctly. Typically, the facing pages contain the same rules or exemplars; one to read about and the other to write on.

Different forms of coursebooks may be designed. My coursebook on *Aphasia and Other Neurogenic Language Disorders* (Singular Publishing Group, 1994) illustrates a different kind of coursebook although both share a common feature: students read them as well as write on them. This coursebook is designed to generate good writing skills in students in speech-language pathology. The learning and teaching of writing skills can be frustrating to both the student and the instructor. Instructors know that merely extolling good writing and asking students to read some of the many available books on how to write well are not effective. Teaching writing skills is time- and effort-intensive because, unless students have examples to follow and feedback to use, their skills do not improve. Students have to write, receive feedback, and rewrite. While it does not obviate the need for writing and rewriting, this coursebook makes that task somewhat more practical for both the student and the instructor.

This coursebook is designed with the following assumptions:

- It is not necessary to have students memorize the rules of grammar to write well
- Students should have many examples of the skills they are expected to learn
- Students should read an exemplar and write one immediately
- Students should write multiple exemplars
- Given exemplars and the student writing should go hand-in-hand
- To the extent possible, students should receive feedback in the classroom itself

How This Coursebook May Be Used

This book has three parts. Part A is designed to teach some basic writing skills that are a foundation for any type of good writing. Part B is designed to teach scientific writing, mostly according to the fourth edition of the *Publication Manual of the American Psychological Association* (1994) (the APA style). Part C helps teach professional writing, including assessment reports, treatment plans, progress reports, and professional correspondence.

Both clinical supervisors and academic course instructors may use this book to teach scientific and professional writing skills. The book may be used in the following contexts:

- A course on writing
- Courses on assessment and diagnosis
- Courses on research methods and introduction to graduate studies
- Clinical practicum and internships
- Independent studies in writing skills
- Informally assigned work to help individual students master good writing skills

A course taught over a semester or quarter offers the most effective context in which to use this book. However, students enrolled in clinical practicum and courses on research methods will find many opportunities to practice technical and professional writing skills in the book. Also, the book is written in such a way as to help implement independent studies and informal writing assignments that are designed to remediate student-specific deficiencies in writing. The book or parts of the book may be assigned to students who complete the writing assignments shown on the right-hand pages. Multiple exemplars and boxed prompts on the right-hand pages reduce mistakes.

Giving Feedback to Students

Through multiple exemplars and assignments, the book itself gives feedback to the student. Still, the instructor should give as much feedback as possible. A problem instructors face is to find time to read large amounts of writing from a big class and give student-specific feedback. This problem may be overcome by having the students complete the writing assignments on the right-hand pages before they come to class. In each class period, all students read aloud at least some portions of their writing. The instructor then gives immediate verbal feedback and all students make corrections on their writing. The instructor makes sure that every student reads some portion of his or her writing and that all students take the feedback seriously. When this method is used the instructor may read only the tests given to the students. Nonetheless, the instructor will have given student-specific feedback on writing. In this method, the instructor spends most, if not all, of the time in class periods on giving feedback to students on their writing. This contrasts with the traditional method of teaching writing in which most of the time is spent on lecturing about rules of writing. The instructor can collect the books from the students one to two times during a semester to make sure that students have completed their writing assignments on the right-hand pages. It is hoped that this coursebook method of teaching will facilitate more writing from students and more feedback from instructors while still keeping both to a manageable level.

A Note on Style Variations

It is helpful to point out to the students that the clinical writing does not follow all aspects of the APA style described in the earlier sections of this book. It also should be pointed out that clinical writing lacks standards that are common for scientific and professional writing. Therefore, clinical reports in this book vary from the APA style in several respects and from each other to show different formats clinicians use.

Clinical reports may use different margins, paragraph styles, indentations, and phrases (incomplete sentences), and one-sentence paragraphs. Most of these may contradict the APA style requirement. However, most other principles of good writing enumerated in the earlier sections apply to clinical writing.

PART A

FOUNDATIONS OF SCIENTIFIC AND PROFESSIONAL WRITING

A.1. BASIC RULES OF USAGE

A.1.1. Do Not Turn a Plural into a Possessive

(Do not use an unnecessary apostrophe.)

Incorrect	Correct	Note
The *characteristic's* of aphasia are well known.	The *characteristics* of aphasia are well known.	A common mistake
The *characteristics'* of aphasia are well known.		
In the *1970's*, the clinicians began to treat language disorders.	In the *1970s*, the clinicians began to treat language disorders.	
I selected 10 *subjects'* on the basis of selection criteria.	I selected 10 *subjects* on the basis of selection criteria.	
The *patients'* have rights.	The *patients* have rights.	

A.1.2. Do Not Turn a Possessive into a Plural

(Use an apostrophe when needed.)

Incorrect	Correct	Note
The *patients* resistance to treatment was high.	The *patient's* resistance to treatment was high.	Singular possessives
The *clients* prognosis is good.	The *client's* prognosis is good.	
The *clinicians* motivation to treat is an important variable.	The *clinicians'* motivation to treat is an important variable.	Plural possessives
The *subjects* socioeconomic background did not have an effect.	The *subjects'* socioeconomic background did not have an effect.	

A.I. BASIC RULES OF USAGE

A.I.I. Do Not Turn a Plural into a Possessive

(Do not use an unnecessary apostrophe.)

Incorrect	Write Correctly
Patients' with dysarthria will have a history of neurologic involvement.	
Many factors' affect the treatment outcome.	
The problems of the 80's will persist into the 90's.	
The clients are in their 60's.	
I studied several variables' related to the subjects' language skills. *Hint: Contains one plural and one possessive.*	

A.I.2. Do Not Turn a Possessive into a Plural

(Use an apostrophe when needed.)

Incorrect	Write Correctly
I will train this clients mother in response maintenance.	
Poorly drawn stimulus pictures can reduce a treatments effectiveness.	
The treatment settings influence cannot be ignored. *Hint: Contains a plural possessive.*	
Several clients progress was slow.	
Clinicians should discuss all of their patients feelings toward treatment.	
We should increase pediatricians awareness of early language problems.	

Hint: Some examples contain a plural and a possessive.

A.1.3. Use the Correct Forms of Possessive Nouns

Several rules dictate the use of a variety of possessive forms. The simplest rule is to add the apostrophe and an *s*, as in *the man's hat, the girl's shoes,* and *cat's tail.* Mistakes arise from the variable practice of adding or not adding 's to words that end in *s*.

Incorrect	Correct	Note
The *boys's* room is large.	The *boys'* room is large.	Most regular plural words do not take an extra *s*; they only have an apostrophe.
The *ladies's* purses are small.	The *ladies'* purses are small.	
The *tigers's* look is ferocious.	The *tigers'* look is ferocious.	
The *mens* health history was not reported.	The *men's* health history was not reported.	Most irregular plurals take 's
The *childrens* ages were not specified.	The *children's* ages were not specified.	
Those *womens* language skills are superior.	Those *women's* language skills are superior.	
The *oxens* hoofs are short.	The *oxen's* hoofs are short.	
The *horse'* skin is shiny.	The *horse's* skin is shiny.	Most words that end in s also take 's.
The *mouse'* tail is long.	The *mouse's* tail is long.	
This one is for old *times's* sake.	This one is for old *times'* sake.	However, a few words that end in s (sound) do not take an extra *s*.
He did it for *appearances's* sake.	He did it for *appearance'* sake.	
Charles' wedding was a grand event.	*Charles's* wedding was a grand event.	Most monosyllabic or disyllabic proper names that end in s, also take 's; a common mistake is to omit the s after the apostrophe.
Mr. *Burns'* humor is wonderful.	Mr. *Burns's* humor is wonderful.	
James' novels are serious.	*James's* novels are serious.	
Thomas' acting is superb.	*Thomas's* acting is superb.	
Keats' poetry is beautiful.	*Keats's* poetry is beautiful.	

A.I.3. Use the Correct Forms of Possessive Nouns

Incorrect	Write Correctly
The boys's boots are here.	
The ladies's dresses are sold here.	
The mens educational status was unknown.	
The childrens language skills were not described.	
Womens professions are constantly changing.	
The horse' speed is unmatched.	
The mouse' manners are awful.	
Have one for old times's sake.	
She would not do it for appearances's sake.	
Charles' graduation party was enjoyable.	
Mr. Burns' 100th birthday celebration was cancelled.	
James' writings are philosophical.	
Thomas' lecture was boring.	
Keats' poetry is immortal.	

Correct Forms of Possessive Nouns *(continued)*

Incorrect	Correct	Note
Jesus's story is moving.	*Jesus'* story is moving.	Longer proper names or names that end with *ses*, that, when combined with 's, are awkward to pronounce, take only an apostrophe.
Moses's ten commandments are well known.	*Moses'* ten commandments are well known.	
Xerxes's army destroyed Athens.	*Xerxes'* army destroyed Athens.	
Demosthenes's pebbles are those in the mouth of a person who stutters.	What are *Demosthenes'* pebbles?	
Plato was *Socrates's* famous pupil.	Plato was *Socrates'* famous pupil.	
The *Browns's* house is large.	The *Browns'* house is large. (Correct: Browns's *shoes are large.*)	Only the apostrophe is used to form possessives in the case of plural forms of family names.
The *Thomas's* cars were stolen.	The *Thomas'* cars were stolen. (Correct: Thomas's *car was stolen.*)	

Correct Forms of Possessive Nouns *(continued)*

Incorrect	Write Correctly
Jesus's kindness was boundless.	
Moses's laws are ancient.	
Xerxes's was a Persian empire.	
What are Demosthenes's pebbles?	
The dialogue was Socrates's teaching method.	
The Jones's hospitality is wonderful.	
The Thomas's vacation was cut short.	

Correct Forms of Possessive Nouns *(continued)*

Incorrect	Correct	Note
We went to *Tom's* and *Jerry's* Pizza Place.	We went to *Tom and Jerry's* Pizza Place. *(Two owners of the place.)*	In the case of group possession, only the last name takes the 's.
We will *take Jim's* and *Jean's* car.	We will take *Jim and Jean's* car. *(Two owners of the same car.)*	
Lent's and *Bent's* book is very interesting.	Lent and Bent's book is very interesting. *(Co-authors of the same book.)*	
We will take *Linda* and *John's* cars.	We will take *Linda's* and *John's* cars. *(Independent owners of two cars.)*	In the case of separate possessions of multiple objects or characteristics, each name takes the 's.
Steinbeck style is different from *Saroyan's.*	*Steinbeck's* style is different from *Saroyan's.* *(Two authors, two styles.)*	
Kent book is interesting, but *Stein's* is boring.	*Kent's* book is interesting, but *Stein's* is boring. *(Two authors, two books.)*	

Correct Forms of Possessive Nouns *(continued)*

Incorrect	Write Correctly
Dean's and Don's Italian restaurant is excellent. *(Two owners of the place.)*	
We borrowed Tom's and Joan's car. *(Two owners of the same car.)*	
Tent's and Nent's book on anatomy is fascinating. *(Co-authors of the same book.)*	
We will take Jim and Kim's vans. *(Independent owners of two vans.)*	
Hemingway style is different from Faulkner's. *(Two authors, two styles.)*	
Knott book has drawings, but Stein's has color pictures. *(Two authors, two books.)*	

A.1.4. Use the Possessive Forms of Pronouns Correctly

The possessive personal pronouns *hers, his, its, ours, yours, theirs,* and *mine* are called *absolute* possessives. Such absolute possessive pronouns, in contrast with other possessives, do not take an apostrophe. Possessive forms of indefinite pronouns, on the other hand, take an apostrophe and *s* ('*s*).

Incorrect	Correct	Note
This book is *her's.*	This book is *hers.*	
This hat is *his'.*	This hat is *his.*	
It's tail is long.	*Its* tail is long.	Do not use an apostrophe to form absolute possessive pronouns.
These are *ours'.*	These are *ours.*	
Isn't she a friend of *your's?*	Isn't she a friend of *yours?*	
This is *their's.*	This is *theirs.*	
That is *mine's.*	That is *mine.*	
Anyones money will do for them.	*Anyone's* money will do for them.	
Who will be the next president is *anybodys* guess.	Who will be the next president is *anybody's* guess.	Use an apostrophe and *s* ('s) to form possessive forms of indefinite pronouns.
Paying taxes is *everyones* responsibility.	Paying taxes is *everyone's* responsibility.	
Someones problems are not his concern.	*Someone's* problems are not his concern.	

A.1.5. Distinguish Contractions from Possessives

Some contracted forms of words should not be confused with possessives.

Incorrect	Correct	Note
They're cat is lost.	*They're* gone now. Their cat is lost.	*They're* is the contracted form of *they are* and *their* is a possessive.
You're office was closed.	*You're* not in your office. Your office was closed.	*You're* is the contracted form of *you are* and *your* is a possessive.
Who's wallet is this?	*Whose* wallet is this?	*Who's* is the contracted form of *who is*; *whose* is the possessive form.

A.1.4. Use the Possessive Forms of Pronouns Correctly

Incorrect	Write Correctly
Is it her's?	
I think it is his'.	
It's mouth is wide.	
Are these ours'?	
I met a friend of your's.	
It may be their's.	
Give me mine's.	
He will take anyones advise.	
He will use anybodys car.	
Taking care of the homeless is everyones responsibility.	
Those ethical concerns are someones problem.	

A.1.5. Distinguish Contractions From Possessives

When appropriate, use the correct contracted form.

Incorrect	Write Correctly
Their in London this summer.	
Your not home tomorrow?	
They're man is not here.	
You're home is big.	
Who's side are you on?	

A.1.6. Use Unusual Singulars and Plurals Correctly

In popular usage, some unusual plurals are accepted as singulars (e.g., *data is* is often seen in print). In scientific and professional writing, these words are used more precisely. Latin plurals can be especially confusing.

Incorrect	Correct	Note
Data *is* presented in Table 1.	Data *are* presented in Table 1.	*Data* is a plural word.
The *datum are* interesting.	The *datum is* interesting.	*Datum* is singular.
The *phenomena* of vocal abuse *is* widespread.	The *phenomenon* of vocal abuse *is* widespread.	*Phenomena* is a plural word.
These *phenomenon have* been recorded.	These *phenomena have* been recorded.	*Phenomenon* is singular.
There is no single *loci* of stuttering.	There is no single *locus* of stuttering.	*Locus* is singular.
The *loci* of stuttering *is* well known.	The *loci* of stuttering *are* well known.	*Loci* is a plural word.
The year of publication should be in *parenthesis*.	The year of publication should be in *parentheses*.	*Parentheses* is plural.
The closing *parentheses is* missing.	The closing *parenthesis is* missing.	The sentence requires the singular *parenthesis*.
I wrote a *theses*.	I wrote a *thesis*.	*Thesis* is singular.
I read *several thesis* before I selected my research topic.	I read *several theses* before I selected my research topic.	*Theses* is plural.
I will sample subjects from the lower socioeconomic *strata*.	I will sample subjects from the lower socioeconomic *stratum*.	*Stratum* is singular.
I will sample subjects from *several* social *stratum*.	I will sample subjects from *several* social *strata*.	*Strata* is plural.
The *papilloma* are benign growths.	*Papillomata* are benign *growths*. A *papilloma* is a benign growth.	*Papillomas* is an accepted plural form, however.
During treatment, I will use a 90% correct criteria.	During treatment, I will use a 90% correct *criterion*.	*Criterion* is singular.
I will use *two criterion* to make the judgment.	I will use *two criteria* to make the judgment.	*Criteria* is plural.
He removed *cortex* from several skulls.	He removed *corteces* from several skulls.	*Cortexes* is an accepted plural.

A.I.6. Use Unusual Singulars and Plurals Correctly

Incorrect	Write Correctly
Her data is quite complex.	
Scientists cannot control many natural phenomenon.	
The phenomena of central auditory processing is a mystery.	
The loci of vocal nodules is variable within a small range.	
Check the closing parentheses of all quotations.	
Put that statement within parenthesis.	
I found no support for that theses.	
All of our thesis are in the library.	
Subjects should be drawn from at least three social stratum.	
The papillomata is benign growth.	

Use Unusual Singulars and Plurals Correctly (continued)

Incorrect	Correct	Note
I found several scholarly *corpus* on the subject.	I found several scholarly *corpora* on the subject.	*Corpora* is plural.
The book has seven *appendix*.	The book has seven *appendixes*.	The APA *Manual* recommends *appendixes;* some other authorities recommend *appendices*.
The author and subject *index* in books are helpful.	The author and subject *indexes* in books are helpful.	The APA *Manual* recommends *indexes;* some other authorities recommend *indices*.
I have *several basis* for my argument.	I have *several bases* for my argument.	*Bases* is plural.
Last semester, I had *many crisis*.	Last semester, I had *many crises*.	*Crises* is plural.
Generally, the term *nucleus* refers to central *cores* of structures.	Generally, the term *nuclei* refers to central *cores* of structures.	*Nuclei* is the plural form of *nucleus*.

Use Unusual Singulars and Plurals Correctly *(continued)*

Incorrect	Write Correctly
Her grading criteria for an A is 90%.	
Good grades and high GRE scores are two criterion for admission.	
Lesion in a single corteces does not prove anything.	
Corpora means a single collection of scholarly writings.	
I found too many appendix in the book.	
He did not have a single bases for his statement.	
I can handle one crises in a semester.	
Generally, the term nuclei refers to a central core of structures.	

A.1.7. Use a Serial Comma

A **serial comma** separates parallel terms in a series. The comma after *men* and before *and* in *women, men, and children* is a serial comma. When you use three or more terms connected with a single conjunction, use a comma after each term that precedes the conjunction. Note that the popular print media does not use a serial comma.

Incorrect	Correct	Note
The child had multiple misarticulations, language delay and a hearing loss.	The child had multiple misarticulations, language delay, and a hearing loss.	The use of conjunction *and*
Our clinicians are intelligent, compassionate and competent.	Our clinicians are intelligent, compassionate, and competent.	
Each token may be exchanged for a sticker, a piece of gum or a small toy.	Each token may be exchanged for a sticker, a piece of gum, or a small toy.	The use of conjunction *or*
Age, education, health, occupation or language skill may be a significant variable in this study.	Age, education, health, occupation, or language skill may be a significant variable in this study.	

A.1.8. Do Not Use a Serial Comma When You Write Only Two Parallel Terms and Connect Them With a Conjunction

Incorrect	Correct	Note
The patient with aphasia had naming, and comprehension problems.	The patient with aphasia had naming and comprehension problems.	
I will recruit both male, and female subjects.	I will recruit both male and female subjects.	In each case, only two terms are joined by a different conjunction (*and, or*)
Plastic tokens, or stickers will be used as reinforcers.	Plastic tokens or stickers will be used as reinforcers.	
The study revealed that age, or prior history of cancer may predict improvement.	The study revealed that age or prior history of cancer may predict improvement.	

A.1.7. Use a Serial Comma

Incorrect	Write Correctly
The training targets will be the correct production of the plural morpheme, the auxiliary and the copula.	
Sensory, neural and sensorineural hearing losses must be distinguished.	
The subjects may chose counseling, syllable prolongation, time-out or response cost as treatment for their stuttering.	
Correct responses will be reinforced with verbal praise, smiles or tokens.	

A.1.8. Do Not Use a Serial Comma When You Write Only Two Parallel Terms and Connect Them With a Conjunction

Incorrect	Write Correctly
The child exhibited omissions, and distortions of several speech sounds.	
An orofacial examination revealed a large tongue, and missing canine teeth.	
The treatment may be started at the word, or the phrase level.	
Aural rehabilitation begins with the selection of an analog, or digital hearing aid.	

A.1.9. Use a Comma to Separate Parenthetic Expressions When You Do Not Use Parentheses

Parenthetic expressions interject an additional idea into a sentence.

Incorrect	Correct
The woman who stuttered though she could not remember it had received treatment before.	The woman who stuttered, though she could not remember it, had received treatment before.
The client who was extremely dysfluent hesitated before starting to read aloud.	The client, who was extremely dysfluent, hesitated before starting to read aloud.
The patient a professional woman in her 50s had a stroke.	The patient, a professional woman in her 50s, had a stroke.
The mean length of utterance when calculated properly can be a good index of early language development.	The mean length of utterance, when calculated properly, can be a good index of early language development.

A.1.10. Place a Comma Before a Conjunction Introducing an Independent Clause

An independent clause can stand alone as a sentence; the terms after the conjunction in the correct example form an independent clause.

Incorrect	Correct
The clinician suggested a treatment program but the client was unresponsive.	The clinician suggested a treatment program, but the patient was unresponsive.
The man was diagnosed with aphasia and the prognosis for recovery was poor.	The man was diagnosed with aphasia, and the prognosis for recovery was poor.
Standardized tests should be administered properly or they will yield meaningless scores.	Standardized tests should be administered properly, or they will yield meaningless scores.

A.1.9. Use a Comma to Separate Parenthetic Expressions When You Do Not Use Parentheses

Incorrect	Write Correctly
The child with misarticulations even though socially competent was not doing well in the school.	
The client who had a severe form of aphasia could not readily respond when asked to name objects.	

A.1.10. Place a Comma Before a Conjunction Introducing an Independent Clause

Incorrect	Write Correctly
The client's mother was asked to attend all treatment sessions but her attendance was poor.	
The students were asked to make oral presentations but their reactions were negative.	
The teacher cooperated with the clinician and the children benefited.	
The father conducted treatment sessions at home and the progress was excellent.	

A.1.11. Join Independent Clauses With a Semicolon When the Clauses Are Not Joined by a Conjunction

The two independent clauses may be rewritten as two separate sentences.

Incorrect	Correct
Stuttering is a speech problem, it should not be ignored.	Stuttering is a speech problem; it should not be ignored.
	Stuttering is a speech problem. It should not be ignored.
Dysphagia can create serious concerns, it can be life-threatening.	Dysphagia can create serious concerns; it can be life-threatening.
	Dysphagia can create serious concerns. It can be life-threatening.
Language disorders can lead to poor academic performance, they should be promptly treated.	Language disorders can lead to poor academic performance; they should be promptly treated.
	Language disorders can lead to poor academic performance. They should be promptly treated.

A.1.12. Use a Dash to Set Off an Abrupt Break or Interruption

Note: The APA *Manual* suggests typing two dashes (--). However, with a computer word processor, you can type an *em-dash* that will be printed as an unbroken line. The examples in this book are em-dashes.

Incorrect	Correct
The speech discrimination test, a standard portion of any audiological diagnostic evaluation revealed no significant problem.	The speech discrimination test—a standard procedure of any audiological diagnostic evaluation—revealed no significant problems.
The administration of a pure probe, if it is administered at all requires much prior work.	The administration of a pure probe—if it is administered at all—requires much prior work.
Response rates recorded at home, although their reliability may be questioned, help document response maintenance.	Response rates recorded at home—although their reliability may be questioned—help document response maintenance.

Note: There is no space separating the dashes (or em-dashes) and the word that precedes or follows it (unless the dash is printed at the end of a line).

A.1.11. Join Independent Clauses With a Semicolon When the Clauses Are Not Joined by a Conjunction

Alternately, write them as two separate sentences.

Incorrect	Write Correctly
Dementia is a neurologically based language disorder, it often is undetected in many nursing homes.	1. 2.
Early treatment of stuttering is effective, this is unknown to some clinicians.	1. 2.
Articulation disorders may persist in some children, they should be promptly treated.	1. 2.
Language acquisition is an interesting subject, I might do a thesis on it.	1. 2

A.1.12. Use a Dash to Set Off an Abrupt Break or Interruption

Incorrect	Write Correctly
Modeling the target response, a basic procedure in language treatment, will be used whenever the client does not imitate.	
Treatment of stuttering, unless the clinician is an ardent believer in spontaneous recovery, should be started as early as possible.	
The incidence of noise-induced hearing loss, a hazardous but controllable by-product of civilization, is on the increase.	

A.1.13. Agreement

Subject and verb should agree in number.
The terms that intervene between the noun phrase and the verb do not affect agreement.

Incorrect	Correct	Note
No single dysfluency *type*—prolongations, interjections, or word repetitions—*justify* diagnosis.	No single dysfluency *type*—prolongations, interjections, or word repetitions—*justifies* diagnosis.	No single dysfluency *type justifies* diagnosis.
She is one of *those* clinicians who *is* always prepared for her sessions.	She is one of *those* clinicians who *are* always prepared for their sessions.	*clinicians* who *are*
For many reasons, the stuttering *person* believes that *they* cannot be treated.	For many reasons, the stuttering *person* believes that *he* or *she* cannot be treated. or For many reasons, stuttering *persons* believe that *they* cannot be treated.	stuttering person believes that *he* or *she* stuttering *persons* believe that
Each *individual* is responsible for their actions.	Each *individual* is responsible for *his* or *her* actions.	*Individual* for *his* or *her*
The *patient*, who has had several years of treatment with no benefit, should have known that *they* are wasting money.	The *patient*, who has had several years of treatment with no benefit, should have known that *she* is wasting money.	The *patient is*
A responsible *student* knows that *they* should study hard.	A responsible *student* knows that *he* (or, he or she) should study hard.	A *student* takes a singular pronoun
These *techniques*, when used appropriately by a competent clinician, is known to be effective.	These tech*niques*, when used appropriately by a competent clinician, *are* known to be effective.	*Techniques are* known to

A.1.13. Agreement

Incorrect	Write Correctly
A disorder of articulation— whether it contains a few or many misarticulations—indicate a need for treatment.	
Naming problems, along with agrammatism, characterizes some patients with aphasia.	
He is one of those individuals who is always late.	
A client who thinks that the clinician should do everything may not take responsibility for their progress.	
Every person has a right to decide on where they want to live.	
Each subject should be told what they will be expected to do during an experiment.	
The clinician who is knowledgeable about accountability knows that they should document client progress.	
Tokens, when dispensed immediately for a correct response, increases the rate of progress.	
Percent dysfluency rates, along with the frequency of each dysfluency, is presented in Table 1.	

Agreement *(continued)*

Incorrect	Correct	Note
Error *scores*, along with the correct score, *was* used in the analysis.	Error *scores*, along with the correct score, *were* used in the analysis.	Error *scores were* used
Every child and adult *go* through the same procedure.	*Every* child and adult *goes* through the same procedure.	A singular verb is used when *every* or *each* precedes a compound subject joined by *and*.
Each man and woman *consider* whether it is right.	*Each* man and woman *considers* whether it is right.	
Either verbal praise *or* informative feedback *are* combined with modeling.	*Either* verbal praise *or* informative feedback *is* combined with modeling. (singular)	When two subjects are linked by *or, either/or,* or *neither/nor,* the verb must be plural if both the subjects are plural and singular if both the subjects are singular.
Either words *or* morphemes *is* appropriate for calculating MLUs.	*Either* words *or* morphemes *are* appropriate for calculating MLUs. (plural)	
Neither he *nor* she *were* interested in the proposal.	*Neither* he *nor* she *was* interested in the proposal. (singular)	
Neither the stimuli *nor* the response consequences *was* well planned.	*Neither* the stimuli *nor* the response consequences *were* well planned. (Plural)	
Neither the treatments *nor* the result *are* replicable.	*Neither* the treatments *nor* the result *is* replicable.	When a singular and a plural subject are linked by *neither/nor, either/or,* or *not only/but also,* the verb form is determined by the subject that is nearer to it.
Either the tokens *or* the verbal praise *are* appropriate.	*Either* the tokens *or* the verbal praise *is* appropriate.	
Not only the treatment procedure, *but also* the treatment *settings, tends* to have an effect on the client's progress.	*Not only* the treatment procedure, *but also* the treatment *settings, tend* to have an effect on the client's progress.	

Agreement *(continued)*

Incorrect	Write Correctly
Every client and the selected family member receive training in recognizing the target response.	
Either time-out or response cost for incorrect responses are combined with positive reinforcement for correct responses.	
Neither the procedure nor the outcome were clearly described.	
Neither the client nor his parents was interested in treatment.	
Neither stutterings nor the phonological processes is reliably measured without training.	
Either verbal feedback or tokens is given to the client for her correct responses.	
Not only the client, but also his colleagues, tends to take the clinician's suggestion seriously.	
The clinician and the client's sister was in the same treatment room.	
Who says "rock 'n' roll are for the devils?"	
Both of us is willing to do it.	
Several of the group is unhappy.	
Some of this mess are your responsibility.	
Some of these effects is unexplained.	

Agreement *(continued)*

Incorrect	Correct	Note
Mother *and* child was interviewed together.	Mother *and* child were interviewed together.	Compound subjects joined by *and* have plural verbs.
Who says *"country and western"* are dead?	Who says *"country and western"* is dead?	Expressions containing *and* that suggest a single concept use singular verbs. *Country and western* is a single concept, although joined by *and*.
Both of us *is* busy.	*Both* of us *are* busy.	A few indefinite pronouns (*both, many, several, few, others*) are always plural and take plural verbs.
Either of them *are* acceptable.	*Either* of them *is* acceptable.	Most other indefinite pronouns (*another, anyone, everyone, each, either, neither, anything, everything, something,* and *somebody*) are singular and take singular verbs.
Some of *this* effect *are* understandable.	Some of *this* effect *is* understandable.(singular)	Some indefinite pronouns (*some, all, none, any, more,* and *most*) can be singular or plural. The verb form is singular or plural depending on the noun the pronoun refers to.
Some of *these* effects *is* understandable.	Some of *these* effects *are* understandable. (plural)	
The *group were* tested in a single session.	The *group was* tested in a single session.	Collective nouns can take singular verbs (if they refer to a single unit) or plural verbs (if they refer to individuals or elements of that unit.)
Seven *individuals* in the group *was* retested.	Seven *individuals* in the group *were* retested.	
The majority were against the idea. A *majority* of people *was* against the idea.	*The majority was* against the idea. A *majority* of people *were* against the idea.	*The majority* is singular; *a majority of people* is plural.

Agreement (continued)

Incorrect	Write Correctly
The experimental group were treated.	
Four subjects in the control group was dropped from the study.	
Either verbal feedback or tokens is given to the client for her correct responses.	
Either family support or teacher support are essential for maintenance of target behaviors in a child.	
Neither the parents nor the grandparents was cooperative.	
Not only the rate of speech, but also the syllable prolongations determines fluency in persons who stutter.	
None of the children is improving with this procedure.	
None of the effect are due to treatment.	
The twin pair were tested in a single session.	
The majority do not agree.	
Politics are full of scoundrels.	
The subjects in the group was tested once.	
The majority were unimpressed.	
A majority of clinicians tends to use this procedure.	

Agreement *(continued)*

Incorrect	Correct	Note
The *news are* bad.	The *news is* bad.	Some words that are typically in the plural form still take singular verbs.
Statistics are an exciting field.	*Statistics is* an exciting field.	
Economics are an inexact science.	*Economics is* an inexact science.	
Statistics shows that the prevalence of phonological disorders in the preschool children is high.	*Statistics show* that the prevalence of phonological disorders in the preschool children is high.	When the word *statistics* refers not to the subject but to some numbers, it takes the plural.
UFO *is* always an exciting *phenomena*.	UFO *is* always an interesting *phenomenon*.	*Phenomenon* is singular and *phenomena* is plural.
They offered *many thesis*, but none too exciting.	They offered *many theses*, but none too exciting.	*Theses* is plural, *thesis* is singular.
I did not think that his *data was* convincing.	I did not think that his *data were* convincing.	*Data* is plural and *datum* is singular.

Agreement *(continued)*

Incorrect	Write Correctly
The local news tend to focus on crime and fire.	
Statistics are not an easy subject.	
Statistics are one of the two courses I took this semester.	
The phenomenon of earthquakes are not well understood.	
It is a scary natural phenomena.	
My theses is as good as yours.	
The theses offered to explain language acquisition does not interest me.	
His data is a bit confusing.	
The datum are enlightening.	

A.1.14. Use Modifiers Correctly

To avoid confusion in the use of modifiers, keep the related words together. This is pointed out in the third column.

Incorrect	Correct	Note
The author and her assistants tested the hearing of all subjects using the procedure described earlier.	The author and her assistants, using the procedure described earlier, tested the hearing of all subjects.	Who used the procedure? Not the subjects!
Distant and mysterious, he stared at the sky.	He stared at the distant and mysterious sky.	Who was mysterious and distant? Not he!
Several additional effects are observed using this technique in clients.	Several additional effects are observed in clients using this technique.	Who observed effects in whom?
Using the standard procedure, the subjects were screened for hearing problems by the experimenter.	Using the standard procedure, the experimenter screened the subjects for hearing problems.	Who used the standard procedure?
The study merely provided a partial support for the hypothesis.	The study provided merely a partial support for the hypothesis.	Place the following modifiers immediately before the words they modify: *almost, only, even, hardly, merely, nearly, exactly, scarcely, just,* and *simply.*
Establishing the target behaviors in the clinic without concern for maintenance is hardly sufficient.	It is hardly sufficient to establish the target behaviors in the clinic without concern for maintenance.	
Limiting children's language assessment to an administration of standardized tests is simply not appropriate.	It simply is not appropriate to limit children's language assessment to an administration of standardized tests.	
Several problems have been observed using negative reinforcement.	Several problems have been observed when clinicians used negative reinforcement.	*Using negative reinforcement* is a dangling modifier because it has no head word.

A.1.14. Use Modifiers Correctly

Incorrect	Write Correctly
The clinician treated stuttering persons using the syllable stretching procedure.	
Consistent with other studies, Smith and Smith (1993) found that cochlear implants are beneficial. Hint: What were consistent? Results or the authors?	
Using the Utah Test, the children's language was screened by the experimenter.	
The treatment only was partially effective.	
He said he was leaving, in a thundering voice.	
The client only had three tokens. (The client had nothing other than three tokens.)	Rewrite the sentence to mean that the client had *no more than* three tokens.
Using tokens, the child was reinforced.	Rewrite to include a person who reinforced the child.
To get a better grade, a long paper was written.	Rewrite the sentence in the active voice and include a subject (e.g., a person's name).
The lecture was made interesting by including videos and computer programs.	Rewrite in the active voice and include a subject.

A.1.15. Do Not Use Pronouns Whose Referents Are Not Clear

Incorrect	Correct	Note
I will use toys and pictures as stimuli, and give reinforcers for correct responses. *They* will be employed only when the response rate does not increase.	I will use toys and pictures as stimuli and give reinforcers for correct responses. *These reinforcers* will be employed only when the response rate does not increase.	*They* refers to what? Correct responses or reinforcers?
A lesion in Broca's area in the left frontal cortex causes Broca's aphasia. *It* may be diagnosed only after careful examination.	A lesion in Broca's area, in the left frontal cortex, may be diagnosed only after careful examination. *Such a lesion* causes Broca's aphasia.	*What* may be diagnosed? The corrected statement says it is the lesion.
Mark went with John because he did not know the address.	Mark did not know the address, so he went with John.	*Who* did not know the address?
On the bulletin board it says that advising starts this week.	The announcement on the bulletin board says that advising starts this week.	An unclear pronoun *it* is replaced.
The client told the clinician that she was happy.	The client told the clinician, "I am happy."	*Who* was happy?

A.1.16. Do Not Break a Sentence into Two

Incorrect	Correct
Upon subjective evaluation. The client's voice was judged normal.	Upon subjective evaluation, the client's voice was judged normal.
The client finally agreed to be tested. After much coaxing from his wife.	After much coaxing from his wife, the client finally agreed to be tested.
I work with 10 children. All with a severe articulation problem.	I work with 10 children, all with a severe articulation problem.
Many hearing impaired children have delayed oral language. And also may have voice problems.	Many hearing impaired children have delayed oral language and also may have voice problems.
I will select 20 subjects for the experiment. Based on the selection criteria.	Based on the selection criteria, I will select 20 subjects.
My client with dysphagia is improving. Because of the treatment.	Because of the treatment, my client with dysphagia is improving.

A.1.15. Do Not Use Pronouns Whose Referents Are Not Clear

Incorrect	Write Correctly
The treatment procedure will include various stimuli, modeling, and positive feedback. It will be used only when the child does not imitate, however.	
The results of many studies, conducted by several investigators have confirmed this. They indicate that we should program maintenance.	
Clinician went with the supervisor because she did not know the practicum site.	
It says in the campus newspaper that an expert on phonological disorders will be on campus.	
Jane told Joan that she was upset.	

A.1.16. Do Not Break a Sentence into Two

Incorrect	Write Correctly
I will treat 12 children with language disorders. Divided into two groups.	
The child finally began to cooperate. After two sessions of crying.	
I tested the hearing of selected subjects. In a sound-treated room.	
The client made excellent progress. In the final four sessions.	
Three phonological processes were eliminated. All during this semester.	
My advisor told me to register. Early in the semester.	

A.1.17. Do Not Turn an Adjective into a Noun

Incorrect	Correct	Note
The *paraplegic* also has aphasia.	The *patient with paraplegia* also has aphasia.	The incorrect versions put the disability first, not the person. The terms in italics are adjectives, not nouns.
The *aphasic* has naming problems.	The *person with aphasia* has naming problems.	
The *autistic* has echolalia.	The *child with autism* has echolalia.	
The *disabled* will be selected.	*Persons who are disabled* will be selected.	

A.1.18. Do Not Turn a Noun into a Verb

Incorrect	Correct	Note
We will *agendize* this matter for the next meeting.	We will place this matter on the next meeting's agenda.	The popular tendency to *ize* a noun has created many awkward verbs.
The treatment targets will be *prioritized*.	I will make a priority list of treatment targets.	
I *gifted* the book to her.	I gave the book to her as a gift.	
First, I *baselined* the target behaviors.	First, I established baselines of the target behaviors.	
The stuttering person was *therapized* by many clinicians.	1. The stuttering person had received therapy from many clinicians. 2. Many clinicians had treated the stuttering person.	

A.1.17. Do Not Turn an Adjective into a Noun

Incorrect	Write Correctly
The dysarthric has multiple communicative disorders.	
The retarded's language is delayed.	
The hemiplegic has motor speech disorders.	
Many aphasics have naming problems.	
The autistic fails to develop emotional attachment.	

A.1.18. Do Not Turn a Noun into a Verb

Many nouns have accepted verb forms, but too much creativity can result in awkward constructions.

Incorrect	Write Correctly
The couple hosted a dinner party.	
She guested on a TV show.	
It is necessary to baseline behaviors before starting treatment.	
He penciled it into his appointment book.	
She thefted my textbooks.	
We partnershipped with the community.	
Our purpose is now collectivized.	

A.1.19. Use the Proper Case of Pronoun

Incorrect	Correct	Note
Between *you* and *I*	Between *you* and *me*.	
They have invited *you* and *myself*.	They have invited *you* and *me*.	Possessive pronouns *hers*, *theirs*, *ours*, and *its* do not take the apostrophe.
Her's is the big house.	*Hers* is the big house.	
It's tail is too bushy.	*Its* tail is too bushy.	
Its an effective procedure.	*It's* an effective procedure.	In formal writing, do not use this contracted form of *it is*.

A.1.20. Make Sure a Participial Phrase at the Beginning of a Sentence Refers to the Grammatical Subject

A participle is a verbal phrase that can function as an adjective; for example, "*Dropped from the second floor,* the ball bounced around," contains the italicized participial phrase; this verbal phrase, acting as an adjective, refers to *the ball,* the subject of the sentence. When the participial phrase does not refer to the grammatical subject in the sentence, it may be described as *dangling* and sounds ludicrous: "*Dropped from the second floor,* I saw the ball bounce around." In this dangling participial phrase, the person, not the ball, is dropped from the second floor!

Incorrect	Correct	Note
A clinician of great reputation, I asked her to treat the client.	A clinician of great reputation, *she* was asked to treat the client.	Who was of great reputation? Not the speaker, as the incorrect version implies!
On discussing treatment options with the client's family, they responded favorably to the clinician.	On discussing treatment options with the client's family, *the clinician* received favorable responses.	Who discussed and who responded favorably are not clear in the incorrect version.
Being in a fixer-upper condition, I found the house a good bargain.	Being in a fixer-upper condition, the house was a good bargain.	The house, not the speaker, was in a fixer-upper condition.
Critically evaluating the evidence presented, the article provides good insight into language acquisition.	*Critically evaluating the evidence presented,* I found the article to provide good insight into language acquisition.	The reader, not the article, critically evaluated the evidence presented.

A.1.19. Use the Proper Case of Pronoun

Incorrect	Write Correctly
You and myself should complete the assessment.	
He told Tom and I to finish the job.	
Their's is the clinic that specializes in myofunctional therapy.	
Ours' is an old dog.	
Its a convenient test to administer.	

A.1.20. Make Sure a Participial Phrase at the Beginning of a Sentence Refers to the Grammatical Subject

Incorrect	Write Correctly
Inexperienced in the treatment of dysphagia, the treatment goals were thought to be easy to establish. *Hint:* Who was inexperienced?	
Without a friend to study with, the failure was inevitable. *Hint:* Whose failure?	
Without help from parents, maintenance of target behaviors was difficult. *Hint:* Whose maintenance?	
Studying carefully the data presented, the article makes a good contribution to treatment research. *Hint:* Who studied the data carefully?	

A.2. BASIC RULES OF COMPOSITION

A.2.1. Design a Broad Outline of Your Paper

Before you begin to write a paper, an essay, a report, or a book chapter, make a broad outline of it. In making an outline, think of what major topics you want to address in the paper. Type each major topic as a major or Level 1 heading. Study the following example.

Note that the author of the exemplar outline made some brief notes under each of the major topics to be addressed:

Theories of Language Acquisition

Brigitte Lopez

Brief Historical Introduction to the Study of Language

(The study of language is age-old, philosophers have studied it, many disciplines study it, and so forth)

Linguistic Theories of Language Acquisition

(Descriptive linguistics, transformational generative grammar, semantic explanations, and so forth)

Psychological Theories of Language Acquisition

(Behavioral explanations, cognitive explanations, interactive explanations)

Recent Developments in Theoretical Explanations

(Integration of different views, suggestions from cross-cultural studies)

Critical Evaluation of Theories

(Lack of experimental support for most theories]

Summary and Conclusions

(Need for additional research; future directions)

Note: There is no one correct outline for a topic. The first outline usually is modified.

A.2. BASIC RULES OF COMPOSITION

A.2.1. Design a Broad Outline of Your Paper

Select a major academic or clinical topic and design an outline for it. Use the level 1 heading style shown in A.2.1 on the previous page. Show your notes.

A.2.2. Design Headings and Subheadings of Your Paper

Select levels of headings; see B.3.16. for examples.

Use the major headings of your initial outline.

Think of additional headings and subheadings.

Give technical headings.

Prefer the shorter to the longer headings.

Try to have the same number of subheadings under all major headings.

Use those headings in your paper.

Theories of Language Acquisition
Bridgette Lopez

Brief historical introduction to the study of language (untitled)

Linguistic Theories of Language Acquisition

Descriptive Linguistic Theories
Transformational Generative Theories
Generative Semantic Theories
Government and Binding Theory
Recent Linguistic Developments

Psychological Theories of Language Acquisition

Behavioral Theories
Cognitive Theories
Interactional Theories

Recent Developments in Theoretical Explanations

Attempts at Integrating Different Views
Suggestions from Cross-cultural Studies

Critical Evaluation of Theories

Comparative Evaluation of Evidence
Suggestions for Future Research

Summary and Conclusions

References

Note: The example contains only two levels of heading; you may need additional headings (see B.3.16.). Also, the APA *Manual* requires underlining the level 2 headings; however, you may print them in italics.

A.2.2. Design Headings and Subheadings of Your Paper

For the outline you have prepared under A.2.1, design headings and subheadings. Revise your headings and subheadings until you can begin writing.

A.2.3. Write Paragraphs That Express Related Ideas

A paragraph expresses *related* ideas. Each paragraph should be a conceptual unit. Different kinds of information should not be mixed-up in a paragraph.

Incorrect	Correct	Note
The subjects will be 25 hearing impaired children. They will come from middle-class families. The children will be selected from a single school within the local school district. The school will be selected randomly. The parents of the children will have normal hearing. The intelligence of the children will be within normal limits.	The subjects will be 25 hearing impaired children. They will come from middle-class families. ~~The children will be selected from a single school within the local school district. The school will be selected randomly~~. The parents of the children will have normal hearing. The intelligence of the children will be within normal limits. The children will be selected from a single school within the local school district. The school will be selected randomly.	The first paragraph describes the subjects. The stricken sentence introduces a different idea (that of subject selection). This should be told in a separate paragraph.
The client will be seen two times a week in 30-min sessions. The initial target behaviors will be the correct production of five phonemes. In the beginning, the client will be trained on discrete trials. Later, conversational speech will be used to stabilize the production of target phonemes. The parents will be trained to help maintain the production of target phonemes. The initial training procedure will include discrete trials. A picture will be used to evoke the target phonemes in words.	The client will be seen two times a week in 30-min sessions. The initial target behaviors will be the correct production of five phonemes. ~~In the beginning, the client will be trained on discrete trials. Later, conversational speech will be used to train the target phonemes. The parents will be trained to help maintain the production of target phonemes.~~ The initial training procedure will include discrete trials. A picture will be used to evoke the target phonemes in words. In the final stage of treatment, conversational speech will be used to stabilize the production of target phonemes. The parents will be trained to help maintain the production of target phonemes.	The first paragraph is about target behaviors. Intrusive sentences about treatment are stricken. The second paragraph is about the training procedure. A separate paragraph is necessary to describe the final stage of treatment.

A.2.3. Write Paragraphs That Express Related Ideas

Incorrect	Write Correctly
Mr. Garcia reported that he began to notice hearing problems some 5 months ago. His wife agreed that it was about that time that her husband began to turn up the volume of their television. He has always enjoyed good physical health. He has been socially active since his retirement two years ago. Around that time, he began to complain that his wife mumbles her speech. Mr. Garcia is a 65-year-old retired electrician. Reportedly, his hearing problem has worsened during the last three weeks.	

Write a Mixed-up Paragraph	Rewrite It Correctly

A.2.4. Do Not Write Paragraphs That Are Too Long

Break longer paragraphs into shorter ones.

Too Long	About Right	Note
Assessment of Timmy's speech and language will include an orofacial examination, a hearing screening, and administration of the Thompson Vocabulary Test, the Jenson Test of Articulatory Performance, and the Shanks Test of Syntactic Constructions. In addition, an extended conversational speech sample will be recorded. The results of this assessment will be integrated with information obtained through case history, reports from other specialists, and information gathered through interview of Timmy's parents. The client's performance on the selected standardized tests will be analyzed according to the test manuals. The conversational speech samples will be analyzed to determine the accuracy of phoneme productions and language structures. The number of phonemes correctly produced, the number of syntactic structures correctly used, and the number of pragmatic rules appropriately followed also will be determined. Besides, the mean length of utterance will be calculated using the Brown method.	Assessment of Timmy's speech and language behaviors will include an orofacial examination, a hearing screening, and administration of the Thompson Vocabulary Test, the Jenson Test of Articulatory Performance, and the Shanks extended Test of Syntactic Constructions. In addition, an conversational speech sample will be recorded. The results of this assessment will be integrated with information obtained through case history, reports from other specialists, and information gathered through interview of Timmy's parents. The client's performance on the selected standardized tests will be analyzed according to the test manuals. The conversational speech samples will be analyzed to determine the accuracy of phoneme productions and language structures. The number of phonemes correctly produced, the number of syntactic structures correctly used, and the number of pragmatic rules appropriately followed also will be determined. Besides, the mean length of utterance will be calculated using the Brown method.	The long paragraph has been broken into smaller ones, each expressing a set of related ideas.

A.2.4. Do Not Write Paragraphs That Are Too Long

Too Long	Rewrite to Make It About Right
Aural rehabilitation is an extended process in which a hearing impaired person is helped to make use of his or her residual hearing. The process begins with hearing testing, but it does not end with it. The process does not end even with a prescription for, or fitting of, a hearing aid. The purchase of a hearing aid is the beginning of aural rehabilitation. The patient should be first familiarized with the workings of the hearing aid. The patient should learn to change the battery, turn on the aid, adjust the volume, and so forth. The patient should know how to take care of the aid, clean it periodically, and protect it from shock and other hazards. The patient also should know when to take it for service. But even more importantly, the patient should know how to benefit from the aid. Initially, the hearing aid's amplification of sound and noise may irritate the person or cause discomfort. Some patients may get headaches until they get used to the aid's amplified sound. The patient should know how to handle the incoming, amplified signal. The audiologist should teach the client to recognize the meaning of sound the patient can now hear.	

A.2.5. Do Not Write One-sentence Paragraphs

This rule applies to scientific and academic writing. **This rule does not apply to clinical report writing.** For the sake of brevity, clinical reports contain one-sentence paragraphs to specify treatment targets, various criteria, and recommendations. This rule is often broken in popular writing as well.

Inappropriate	Appropriate	Note
The effects of communication disorders are several. The disorders create many social and occupational difficulties. Some persons with communicative disorders may withdraw from normal social interactions. Some employers may be unwilling to hire persons with communicative problems. Persons who have communicative problems may experience certain emotional problems. Such persons may be frustrated in their attempts at communication. People who stutter or those who have aphasia experience frustration when they cannot express themselves promptly.	The effects of communication disorders are several. The disorders create many social and occupational difficulties. Some persons with communicative disorders may withdraw from normal social interactions. Some employers may be unwilling to hire persons with communicative problems. Persons who have communicative problems may experience certain emotional problems. Such persons may be frustrated in their attempts at communication. For example, people who stutter or those who have aphasia experience frustration when they cannot express themselves promptly.	The one-sentence paragraph stands alone with nothing to connect to. Note that when the two paragraphs are combined, some change in the wording may be necessary to provide transition.

A.2.5. Do Not Write One-sentence Paragraphs

Choose an academic topic.

Write Four One-sentence Paragraphs	Integrate the Four One-sentence Paragraphs into a Single Paragraph

A.2.6. Begin and End Most Paragraphs With Transitory Sentences

Lack of transition breaks the flow of thought and confuses the reader. To achieve smooth transition, **do**:

- end and begin adjacent paragraphs with a related idea.
- suggest what will be said in the next paragraph.
- make reference to what was said in the previous paragraph.

However, **do not**:

- introduce new topics abruptly.
- randomly shift topics across paragraphs.

Rough Transition	Smoother Transition	Note
1. Methods of analysis of articulatory errors have undergone many changes. Traditionally, the clinicians have made the sound-by-sound analysis to judge the accuracy of individual sound productions. **2.** In the place-voice-manner analysis, sounds are classified into patterns based on these phonetic features. Errors also are similarly classified. **3.** Phonological processes are simplifications of speech sound productions that help classify multiple errors into groups or patterns. Another approach is that of distinctive feature analysis, which was suggested before the phonological process approach.	**1.** Methods of analysis of articulatory errors have undergone many changes. Traditionally, the clinicians have made the sound-by-sound analysis to judge the accuracy of individual sound productions. Therefore, *there is no attempt to see a pattern in the errors* based on an underlying principle. **2.** The first approach to see a *pattern in the errors* was based on the place-voice-manner analysis. In this approach, sounds are classified into patterns based on the three phonetic features. Therefore, errors also are similarly classified. This classification resulted in somewhat *simplified patterns of errors.* **3.** A method of classification resulting in more *complex patterns of errors* was suggested by the next approach: analysis of the distinctive features of speech sounds. Soon, however, a new approach based on *phonological theories* was proposed. **4.** *Phonological theories* proposed that phonological processes, which are patterned simplifications of speech sound productions, explain errors of articulation. These processes help classify multiple errors into groups or patterns.	The first paragraph of the first column set the stage for a historical view. But with no transition and no historical sense, the second paragraph is isolated.

The first two paragraphs of the second column are related because of the common, italicized words. A theme flows from the first to the second paragraph.

The third paragraph of the first column abruptly introduces the phonological process approach. The rewriting achieves smoother transition as shown by a repeated theme (italicized words in the second and the third paragraphs).

The third paragraph in the first column confuses the historical sequence because of an abrupt shift to phonological approach before mentioning the distinctive feature approach. |

A.2.6. Begin and End Most Paragraphs With Transitory Sentences

Rough Transition	Rewrite With Smoother Transition

College students in the 90s face many problems. A basic problem all college students face is lack of money. In a technological society, everyone needs a college degree to make a decent living. Unfortunately, not everyone can afford the ever-escalating cost of higher education.
    With limited resources, colleges are offering less financial aid to students. The rate at which the cost of higher education has escalated has outpaced that of inflation. This may be due to dwindling state support for higher education.
    Reduced financial aid makes it especially difficult for students with families. Balancing the needs of a family and the demands of an academic program is difficult. The difficulty is aggravated when faced with financial problems. Limited financial aid makes it especially difficult for students with families.
 	
Hint: Each paragraph contains a transitory sentence; only it is misplaced.	

A.2.7. Use the Active Voice

The opposite of active voice is passive voice. In sentences written in active voice, the subject of a verb performs the action (e.g., *the boy hit the ball*); in sentences written in passive voice, the subject of a verb is acted upon or said to receive the action (e.g., *the ball was hit by the boy*). Passive sentences are long and indirect. In most cases, they can be avoided to make writing more direct and easier to understand.

Passive	Preferred Active
The supervisor was the person with whom I spoke.	I spoke to the supervisor.
The children were brought to the clinic by their mothers.	The mothers brought their children to the clinic.
The target responses will be modeled by the clinician.	The clinician will model the target responses.
When the target behaviors are selected, stimulus materials will be prepared.	After selecting the target behaviors, I will prepare the stimulus materials.

A.2.8. Prefer the Shorter to the Longer Sentence Structures

Maintain some variety, however. Alternate longer sentences with shorter ones.

Longer Sentences	Preferred Shorter Sentences	Note
Many clinicians who employ the traditional method of articulation training tend to use nonsense syllables in the early stages of training, along with an emphasis on ear training with a view to promote auditory discrimination of speech sounds.	Many clinicians employ the traditional method of articulation training. In this method, the clinicians use nonsense syllables in the early stages of training. The training emphasis is on the auditory discrimination of speech sounds.	One sentence has been broken into three. These shorter sentences are easier to read and understand.
The many compounding problems of the hearing impaired child include social isolation, academic difficulties, problems in language learning, and many others that when unchecked by a well designed management plan, can lead to additional problems later in life which are then very difficult to manage.	The many compounding problems of the hearing impaired child include social isolation, academic difficulties, and language learning problems. Unless checked by a well designed management plan, these problems can lead to additional difficulties later in life. Such long-standing problems are difficult to manage.	The maze of long sentences obscures a chain of ideas or events. Some long sentences contain unnecessary words that can be cut out to shorten them.

A.2.7. Use the Active Voice

Passive	Rewrite in Preferred Active Terms
Central auditory processing problems may be assessed by various tests.	
The client's behavior problems were not controlled by the clinician.	
There are many procedures that may be used in aural rehabilitation.	
The clinician was upset by the child's uncooperative behavior.	

A.2.8. Prefer the Shorter to the Longer Sentence Structures

Longer Sentences	Rewrite in Shorter Sentences
Many clinicians, who believe that auditory training is an important part of aural rehabilitation of hearing impaired children, nonetheless do not appreciate the need for such training in case of adult hearing impaired individuals, although it is well established that the recognition and discrimination of speech sounds is an integral part of any program of aural rehabilitation designed for individuals of all ages.	
While the psychoanalytic theory has stated that stuttering is due primarily to oral and anal regression during infancy, the behavioral view has asserted that stuttering is due to faulty conditioning, and the neurophysiological theories have implicated either the auditory system with defective feedback loops, the laryngeal mechanism with improper neural control, or the brain with its problems in language processing.	

A.2.9. Use Positive Terms

Instead of saying what it is not, say what it is, even when what is said is negative. Avoid using the word "not" whenever possible. For example, instead of writing, "The client was not happy," write, "The client was unhappy."

Negative	Preferred Positive
The client often did not come to the treatment sessions at the appointed time.	The client often came late to treatment sessions.
These treatment procedures are not very effective.	These treatment procedures are ineffective.
The results of our tests do not suggest that the client does not have central auditory processing problems.	The results of our tests suggest that the client has central auditory processing problems.
I do not believe that the client does not have a phonological disorder.	The client has a phonological disorder.
I do not think that these procedures will not work with aphasia.	1. I think that these procedures will work with aphasia. 2. These procedures will work with aphasia.
The man is not honest.	The man is dishonest.
The clinician did not pay any attention to the supervisor's suggestion.	The clinician ignored the supervisor's suggestion.

A.2.10. Avoid Too Many Qualifications

Too many qualifications make your writing timid, weak, and uncertain. The reader will be unsure of what you say. Let your statements be as definite as the *observations or data warrant.*

Overly Qualified and Weak	Stronger and Clearer
It is possible that some clinicians do not have a very strong belief in the validity of this theory.	1. Some clinicians doubt the validity of this theory. 2. Some clinicians reject this theory.
The data may possibly suggest that in at least some cases, the technique may have some limited use.	The data suggest that the technique may be useful in some cases.
It would be beneficial to use this assessment procedure with children though it may or may not be just as effective with adults.	This assessment procedure may be more useful with children than with adults.
It may be possible to use the criterion of 90% correct response rate before dismissing the client.	The dismissal criterion will be 90% correct response rate.

A.2.9. Use Positive Terms

Negative	Rewrite in Preferred Positive Terms
The instructor did not have much confidence in the student's explanation.	
The nativist theory does not do a great job of explaining language acquisition.	
Asking Yes/No questions may not be an effective method of evoking continuous speech from a child.	
Some clinicians believe that phoneme auditory discrimination training may not be an efficient method of treatment.	
Surgical procedures may not be very effective in the rehabilitation of certain types of hearing impairment.	

A.2.10. Avoid Too Many Qualifications

Overly Qualified and Weak	Stronger and Clearer
Theory may be of some value in explaining at least a small aspect of this complex phenomenon.	
I hope that with the help of this new procedure, I may be able to have some effect on the child's communication.	
I am favorably disposed to using the rate reduction procedure in the treatment of stuttering.	
I expect that I may be able to convince the parents that they may consider the possibility of holding informal treatment sessions at home.	
I expect that in all likelihood, the digital hearing aid may prove to be beneficial for this client.	

A.2.11. Use Definite, Specific, and Concrete Language

Avoid the overuse of generalized terms whose meanings are not clear. Be specific in describing symptoms of disorders, behaviors, procedures, effects, services, and so forth.

Incorrect	Correct
In all likelihood, the treatment seems to have had some positive effect on the life of the client.	Possibly, treatment helped the client speak more fluently.
Various visual and auditory stimulus input methods will be used in treatment.	Pictures, objects, action figures, and tape-recorded models of speech sound productions will be used in treatment.
I will make sure that the parents support Johnny's production of target behaviors at home.	I will ask the parents to praise Johnny at home for his correct production of speech sounds.
A variety of grammatic morphemes will be the treatment targets.	Many grammatic morphemes, including the regular plural, possessive, the articles, and prepositions will be the treatment targets.
The child was not very cooperative during assessment.	Often crying or whining, the child refused to name the pictures shown.
A variety of standardized and nonstandardized tests or procedures will be used in assessing the client's language.	Along with a conversational speech sample, the client's language will be evaluated with the Bankson Language Test, the Peabody Picture Vocabulary Test, and the Test for Examining Expressive Morphology.
The child with cleft palate and his or her family need numerous services from an array of different specialists.	The child with cleft palate and his or her family need services from many specialists including pediatricians, dentists, orthodontists, plastic surgeons, otologists, audiologists, speech-language pathologists, psychologists, and others.
Lack of treatment progress had some negative effect on the client's emotionality.	The client was disappointed because of lack of progress in treatment.

Note: In each of the correct examples, such general terms as "a variety of," "various," "numerous," "several," "many," "some," "positive effect," and so forth are replaced by specific terms.

A.2.11. Use Definite, Specific, and Concrete Language

Incorrect	Write Correctly
The man with aphasia did not seem very happy during the treatment sessions. Describe behaviors that suggest unhappiness.	
Voice therapy seems to have changed the life of Mr. Shreik. Describe one or two changes in life.	
I will use any and all means of promoting response maintenance at home. Specify a few techniques.	
The child did not want to be assessed. What did the child do?	
I will use many different procedures to assess the child's articulation. Specify two or three procedures.	
Stuttering has many kinds of effects on most aspects of life. Describe a few effects.	
A hearing impaired child with an active ear pathology needs a variety of professional services from many different specialists. Name a few services and professionals.	
The client was unfavorably disposed to continuing treatment next semester. What did the client say?	

A.2.12. Eliminate or Replace Unnecessary Phrases

To be precise and more effective, eliminate popular but unnecessary words and phrases. While cluttering sentences, they add nothing to the meaning. See the examples on the following pages.

Unnecessary Words	Recommendation
abilities (unless you distinguish it from action)	describe actions
along the lines of	eliminate
as a matter of fact	eliminate
as far as . . . is (are) concerned	eliminate
at the present time	now
at this point in time	now
by means of	eliminate
call your attention to the fact that	remind you or notify you
due to the fact that	eliminate
experienced an inability	describe actions
experienced great difficulty	describe actions
for all intents and purposes	eliminate
hands-on experience	experience
I was unaware of the fact that	I did not know
in any shape or form	eliminate
in order to	to
in spite of the fact that	eliminate
in the time frame	in about
in the area of	name the area
in the event that	if
is considered to be	eliminate
on account of the fact that	eliminate
owing to the fact that	eliminate
question as to whether	whether
the fact of the matter is	eliminate
the field of	name the discipline
the type of (unless you describe different types)	eliminate
there is no doubt that	no doubt, doubtless, undoubtedly
this is a subject that	this subject
to tell the truth	just say what you want to say
unable to (in most cases)	describe actions
until such time as	until
used for the purpose of	used for (to)
with regards to	eliminate
with respect to	eliminate
with reference to	eliminate

A.2.12. Eliminate or Replace Unnecessary Phrases

Find at least five unnecessary phrases that people use:

1.

2.

3.

4.

5.

Write sentences containing unnecessary phrases in the first column and their revised forms in the second column.

Imprecise	Precise

Eliminate or Replace Unnecessary Phrases (continued)

Imprecise	Precise
In the time frame of an hour, a complete assessment may be made.	In about an hour, a complete assessment may be made.
Aphasia *is considered to be* a language disorder.	Aphasia is a language disorder.
We have much controversy *in the area of* language treatment.	We have much controversy in language treatment.
Reading, writing, and speaking *abilities* were affected.	Reading, writing, and speaking were affected.
The patient *experienced an inability* to produce speech.	The patient could not produce speech.
The tongue demonstrated weakness *with regards* to lateral strength.	The tongue demonstrated lateral weakness.
A mixed probe will be *the type of probe* administered.	A mixed probe will be administered.
If the client *is unable* to produce the word, the clinician will model it.	If the client cannot produce a word, the clinician will model it.
She *experienced great difficulty* speaking as demonstrated by slow, labored, and effortful speech.	Her speech was slow, labored, and effortful.
For all intents and purposes, assessment and diagnostics mean the same.	Assessment and diagnostics mean the same.
Treatment goals were not achieved *due to the fact that* the client missed several sessions.	Treatment goals were not achieved because the client missed several sessions.
On account of the fact that she was unemployed, she could not afford treatment.	Because she was unemployed, she could not afford treatment.
John won *in spite of the fact that* he was injured.	John won although he was injured.
We cannot offer any monetary rewards *at this point in time*.	We cannot offer any monetary rewards now.
At the present time, my case load is full.	Now my caseload is full.

Eliminate or Replace Unnecessary Phrases *(continued)*

Imprecise	Write Precisely
Modeling may be considered to be an effective stimulus control procedure.	
In the area of phonological disorders, we have many assessment procedures.	
Respiration, phonation, and articulation abilities were disturbed.	
The patient with laryngectomy experiences an inability to phonate normally.	
With regards to long-term effects, loud noise is detrimental to normal hearing.	
A single-subject design will be the type of design to be used in this study.	
When the client is unable to imitate a target response, I will use the shaping procedure.	
He experienced great difficulty in producing phonemes in sequence as demonstrated by his trial-and-error movement of the articulators.	

Eliminate or Replace Unnecessary Phrases *(continued)*

Imprecise	Precise
The question as to whether children with articulation disorders have phonological disorders has been debated.	Whether children with articulation disorders have phonological disorders has been debated.
In the field of communicative disorders	In communicative disorders
He has *the ability to* lead the team.	He can lead the team.
It is good to get some *hands-on* experience in the workplace.	It is good to get some experience in the workplace.
During treatment, improvement *in terms of* the response rates was good.	During treatment, the response rates improved.
As far as the client's correct production of phonemes was concerned, the results were disappointing.	At home, the client did not (does not) correctly produce the phonemes.
In the event that Hector cannot complete the task, Sheila will take over.	If Hector cannot complete the task, Sheila will take over.
We will win *by means of* working harder.	We will win by working harder
He is a man who (*she is a woman who*) knows about religion.	He (She) knows about religion.
The clinician spoke *along the lines of* normal language development.	The clinician spoke about normal language development.
With reference to mild conductive hearing loss in infancy, it may cause language delay.	Mild conductive hearing loss in infancy may cause language delay.
With respect to our earlier conversation, I will see you tomorrow.	As we talked earlier, I will see you tomorrow.
To tell you the truth, I will not be able to attend your party.	I am sorry that I cannot attend your party.
There is no doubt that he will come to the party.	He undoubtedly will come to the party.
I was unaware of the fact that she was going to bring her child.	I did not know that she was going to bring her child.
Owing to the fact that early treatment of language disorders is effective, we recommend immediate treatment to your child.	Because early treatment of language disorders is effective, we recommend immediate treatment to your child.

Eliminate or Replace Unnecessary Phrases *(continued)*

Imprecise	Write Precisely
Morphologic training was not initiated this semester due to the fact that the client did not meet the other targets.	
On account of the fact that they did not attend the IEP meetings, the parents could not be informed about the treatment targets.	
The client made excellent progress in spite of the fact that she had a severe articulation problem.	
The fact of the matter is that many untested theories confuse the clinician.	
Our waiting list is long at this point in time.	
At the present time, all the treatment targets have been achieved.	
Until such time as the interfering behaviors are controlled, language targets cannot be trained.	
Tokens may be used for the purposes of reinforcement.	
In order to assess the client's syntactic structures, a language sample was recorded.	
The researchers have investigated the question as to whether mild conductive hearing impairment in young children causes language delay.	

Eliminate or Replace Unnecessary Phrases *(continued)*

Imprecise	Precise
I am very busy *until such time as* the holidays are over.	I am very busy until the holidays are over.
Our office is *used for the purposes of* distribution.	Our office is used for distribution.
In order to teach the morphologic features, I will model the correct responses.	To teach the morphologic features, I will model the correct responses.
I wish to call your attention to the fact that aphasia treatment is effective.	Please note that aphasia treatment is effective.
This is a subject that interests me.	This subject interests me.

Eliminate or Replace Unnecessary Phrases *(continued)*

Imprecise	Write Precisely
The client has the ability to speak fluently.	
You can get some hands-on experience in word processing at our computer lab.	
In terms of making a complete assessment, language samples are excellent.	
As far as the client's motivation for treatment is concerned, you should make a good judgment.	
In the time frame of 20 minutes, you should administer a probe.	
In the event that the treatment sessions cannot be held twice a week, a once-a-week schedule might be tried.	
Articulation was assessed by means of the Goldman-Fristoe Test of Articulation.	
She is a clinician who can treat patients with aphasia.	
The clinician worked along the lines of response maintenance.	
The field of audiological practice is challenging and stimulating.	
I was unaware of the fact that the client had prior therapy.	
Owing to the fact that the child has a hearing loss, there may be language delay.	
I wish to call your attention to the fact that the patient may have suffered head injury.	
This is a subject that I am interested in doing a thesis on.	

A.2.13. Avoid Redundant Phrases

Most redundant phrases contain two or more words that mean the same. Eliminate these words.

Redundant	Essential
future prospects	prospects
advance planning	planning
absolutely incomplete	incomplete
exactly identical	identical
repeat again	again
each and every	each *or* every
totally unique	unique
uniquely one of a kind	one of a kind *or* unique
reality as it is	reality
actual facts solid facts true facts	facts
famous and well-known	famous *or* well-known
goals and objectives (when the two are not distinguished)	goals *or* objectives; *or,* distinguish the two
three different kinds	three kinds
seven different varieties	seven varieties
four different types	four types
as of yet	yet
prison facilities church facilities hospital facilities	prison, church, hospital
crisis situation	crisis
problem situation	problem
prepay first	prepay *or* pay first
free gift	gift *or* free
positive growth	growth
bad weather conditions deteriorating economic conditions deteriorating client response conditions	bad weather deteriorating economy client's deteriorating responses
positive affirmative action	affirmative action
actively involved, actively looking	involved, looking
preconditions	conditions
unexpected surprise	surprise
successfully completed successfully avoided	completed avoided
make an effort to try	make an effort *or* try
advice and counsel	advice *or* counsel
necessary and essential	necessary *or* essential
fair and equitable	fair *or* equitable

A.2.13. Avoid Redundant Phrases

Find five redundant phrases used in everyday language. Suggest the essential terms.

Redundant Phrases	Essential

Avoid Redundant Phrases *(continued)*

Redundant Phrases	Essential
The *future prospects* of speech-language pathology are excellent.	The future of speech-language pathology is excellent.
NSSLHA held an *advanced planning* meeting for fund raising.	NSSLHA held a planning meeting for fund raising.
The story was *absolutely incomplete.*	The story was incomplete.
The student's plagiarized paper was *exactly identical* to the author's.	The student's plagiarized paper was identical to the author's.
Can you *repeat* that *again?*	Can you repeat that?
Each and every student was required to write a paper.	Each (*or,* Every) student was required to write a paper.
Each client is *totally unique.*	Each client is unique.
This new test on traumatic brain injury is *uniquely one of a kind.*	This new test on traumatic brain injury is one of a kind (*or,* unique).
Out in the world, *reality as it is,* is different from what the professors' imagine.	Out in the world, reality is different from what the professors' imagine.
Language Acquisition Device (LAD) is a *true fact* of language development.	Language Acquisition Device is a fact of language development.
She is a *famous and well-known* lecturer.	She is a famous (*or,* well-known) lecturer.
We should write some *goals and objectives.* Note: This is fine when goals are distinguished from objectives. When they are not, the phrase is redundant.	We should write some goals (*or,* objectives).
We have *three different kinds* of language tests.	We have three kinds of language tests.
It is not done *as of yet.*	It is not done yet.
We will visit the *prison facilities.*	We will visit the prison.
We have a *crisis situation* on hand.	We have a crisis on hand.
Deteriorating client *response conditions* were distressing.	Deteriorating client responses were distressing.
There were some *preconditions* for negotiation.	There were some conditions for negotiation.

Avoid Redundant Phrases (*continued*)

Redundant Phrases	Essential
The future prospects of maintenance of fluency are excellent.	
The officers held an advanced planning meeting.	
The treatment report was absolutely incomplete.	
The two stimuli used on treatment and probe trials were exactly identical.	
The clinician will repeat modeling again.	
Each and every client's family members should be trained in response maintenance.	
For each client, we do not need totally unique treatment procedures.	
I found uniquely one of a kind software for surfing the internet.	
Reality as it is may be more disappointing than we imagine it to be.	
An actual fact of clinical practice is some degree of apprehension.	
He is a famous and well-known author.	
My treatment goals and objectives were not clear.	

Avoid Redundant Phrases (continued)

Redundant Phrases	Essential
She is *actively looking* for a job.	She is looking for a job.
We had an *unexpected surprise* in therapy session.	We had a surprise in therapy session.
She *successfully completed* our graduate program.	She completed our graduate program.
The person who stutters *successfully avoids* certain words.	The person who stutters avoids certain words.
I will make an *effort to try* to train parents in response maintenance.	I will try to train parents in response maintenance.
A *necessary and essential* element of treatment is positive reinforcement.	A necessary (*or,* essential) element of treatment is positive reinforcement.
The grading was *fair and equitable.*	The grading was fair (*or,* equitable).

Avoid Redundant Phrases (*continued*)

Redundant Phrases	Essential
We have three different types of assignments in the class.	
We offer 11 different varieties of language treatment.	
The treatment program is not complete as of yet.	
We will visit the hospital facilities.	
The problem situation is getting worse.	
The bad weather conditions were getting worse.	
I did not accept their preconditions for employment.	
My client is actively involved in the treatment process.	
The child's sudden temper tantrum was an unexpected surprise to me.	
The client successfully completed all steps in the treatment.	
She made an effort to try to keep the appointment.	
Paper work is a necessary and essential element of professional practice.	
The pay raise offered to us was fair and equitable.	

A.2.14. Avoid Wordiness

Wordiness is the use of many kinds of words that makes the writing vague, timid, and unnecessarily long.

Wordy	Precise	Note
It seems to me that it certainly is very important to consider many factors in selecting treatment procedures for my clients.	I should consider many factors in selecting treatment procedures for my clients.	It is assumed that you will soon specify at least a few factors.
It became evident from my conversation with the parents of the child that they had a very difficult time to do what they were told to do because of their busy life style.	The parents of the child told me that they did not have time to conduct treatment sessions at home.	
Although the client was certainly not negatively disposed to continuing the treatment for a reasonable amount of time, she finally decided to discontinue it.	The client discontinued the treatment, although she said she wanted to continue it.	The overused word *certainly* often suggests no certainty.
There were several crucial factors that led me to select these assessment procedures.	These assessment procedures were selected because of their known reliability, validity, and simplicity.	Often, the word *crucial* is an overstatement.
A variety of procedures will be used.	Many procedures will be used.	Procedures may be specified in subsequent sentences.
A number of clients were treated.	Several clients were treated.	It is assumed that the exact number is unimportant.
Certain limitations of standardized tests make it imperative to carefully reconsider the whole issue of reliability and validity of assessment procedures.	Because of the limitations of standardized tests, we should reconsider the reliability and validity of assessment procedures.	Limitations will have been specified.
It is not in the least inappropriate to offer the suggestion that cochlear implant may be a reasonably attractive method of aural rehabilitation that should not be rejected out of hand.	The option of cochlear implant should be considered.	The more precise statement says it positively as well.

A.2.14. Avoid Wordiness

Wordy	Rewrite Precisely
In my judgment, it is reasonable to conclude that there are different types of aphasia although many symptoms are common to the different types.	
I personally think that it is not totally inappropriate to suggest that children with multiple misarticulations have a phonological disorder.	
I used two tests which were known to have a reasonable degree of reliability.	
It certainly seems to me that we need more treatment efficacy research.	
A variety of investigators have found it appropriate to suggest that both genetic and environmental factors play a causative role in stuttering.	
It is not unreasonable to suggest that we carefully consider all minimally attractive alternatives available to us as at this important juncture.	
It is certainly apparent to most competent clinicians that it is reasonably worthwhile to offer voice therapy to certain clients who may wish to consider it as an attractive alternative to surgical procedures.	
If one were to infer from these assessment data that the client has Broca's aphasia, the inference would certainly not seem totally inappropriate.	

A.2.15. Keep Related Words Together

Intervening words that split related words can confuse the meaning. Think which words of a sentence should be adjacent to each other.

Incorrect	Correct	Note
He ate seven hot dogs for lunch last Friday, and three more for dinner.	Last Friday, he ate seven hot dogs for lunch and three more for dinner.	
An unruly behavior of a child, if you do not control it, will prevent rapid progress in treatment.	Unless controlled, a child's unruly behavior will prevent rapid progress in treatment.	What prevents rapid progress?
Treatment of cluttering, because of limited research, is not well established.	Because of limited research, treatment of cluttering is not well established.	What is not well established?
Most clinicians, although they are keenly interested in it, are not well trained in the assessment of dysphagia.	Although they are keenly interested in it, most clinicians are not well trained in the assessment of dysphagia.	In what are the clinicians not well trained?
The supervisor asked clinicians to write a treatment plan for each client at the meeting Wednesday.	At the meeting Wednesday, the supervisor asked clinicians to write a treatment plan for each client.	Not write a treatment plan at the meeting!
This is an assessment report on Mr. Davis, referred to us by Dr. Benson, seen last week in our facility.	This is an assessment report on Mr. Davis, seen last week in our facility. He was referred to us by Dr. Benson.	Dr. Benson was not seen last week!
Women who are pregnant, but unaware of its bad effects, may continue to drink alcohol.	Women who are pregnant, but unaware of the bad effects of alcohol on the fetus, may continue to drink.	Bad effects of drinking or pregnancy?
The human fertility clinic extracted multiple ova from women, then froze them.	The human fertility clinic extracted multiple ova from women. The clinic then froze the ova.	Ova, not women, were frozen!

Note: Misplaced modifiers (see A.1.14.) also create the same kind of problems as splitting related words.

A.2.15. Keep Related Words Together

Incorrect	Write Correctly
Maintenance of target behaviors, if not carefully programmed, will not be achieved.	
In assessing phonological disorders, although many procedures may be appropriate, conversational speech is the most productive.	
Meeting the IEP goals within three months, even if I work hard and the child is regular for sessions, will be difficult.	
The selected target behaviors may be taught, assuming that the client will be regular for treatment sessions, in about 10 sessions.	
The final target of treatment, it has been suggested, is maintenance.	
The treatment procedure will include generalized reinforcers, to make it more effective.	
Clinicians who are inexperienced, but do not know how hazardous it is, may cause serious problems by using wrong methods of dysphagia treatment.	
I wrote this treatment plan for Mrs. Jones, after careful consideration of her strengths and weaknesses.	

A.2.16. Maintain Parallelism

Parallelism is the expression of a series of ideas in the same grammatic form. Parallel forms are forceful and concise. Parallelism is broken when some ideas are expressed in one form and the other, coordinated ideas in different forms.

Incorrect	Correct	Note
Children with language disorders tend to be deficient in their use of grammatic morphemes, syntactic structures, and *they also may have a limited vocabulary.*	Children with language disorders tend to be deficient in their use of grammatic morphemes, syntactic structures, and complex words.	The incorrect versions have a *nonparallel final clause.*
The hearing impaired child has difficulty speaking, reading, and *self-confidence.*	The hearing impaired child has difficulty speaking, reading, and in maintaining self-confidence.	The correct versions restore parallelism to the final clause.
Disadvantages of primary reinforcers include satiation, dietary restriction, and *they also are difficult to administer to groups.*	Disadvantages of primary reinforcers include satiation, dietary restriction, and problematic group administration.	
Parental reinforcement of target behaviors helps maintenance by *not* allowing extinction, strengthening the behaviors, and increasing their use in natural environments.	Parental reinforcement of target behaviors helps maintenance by *not* allowing extinction, by strengthening the behaviors, and by increasing their use in natural environments.	The incorrect version is nonparallel because the word *not* applies only to the first in the series. In the correct version, the repetition of *by* restores parallelism.
Today's treatment objectives include: 1. training the /s/ in the word final positions 2. working on naming skills 3. oral-motor exercises	Today's treatment objectives include: 1. training the /s/ in the word final positions 2. working on naming skills 3. providing oral-motor exercises	Mixture of verb phrases and noun phrases is corrected. A common mistake in numbered or bulleted lists
The targets, the stimuli, and reinforcers, should all be specified.	The targets, the stimuli, and the reinforcers should all be specified.	An article is either repeated before all parallel terms, or is used only before the first term. (The targets, stimuli, and reinforcers . . .)

A.2.16. Maintain Parallelism

Incorrect	Write Correctly
Many persons who stutter have been frustrated in the past because the therapists lacked adequate training, supervised experience, and the therapists' scientific knowledge of stuttering has been limited.	
Persons with communicative problems have difficulty talking, reading, and self-confidence.	
Some of the side effects of saying "No" to a client are aggression, reticence, and the client may also feel resentment toward the clinician.	
To promote response maintenance, I will: • select stimuli from the client's home • train self-monitoring skills • teach target behavior charting • parent training will be included	
Patients with aphasia may be treated with auditory stimulation and verbal expression also may be taught.	
The theory may be criticized for three reasons: first, it is illogical; second, it is nonempirical; third, it is also difficult to apply.	
I trained the parents, the grandparents, siblings, and teachers.	
The client may receive treatment in Fall, Spring, or in Summer terms. *Hint:* The preposition is either repeated before all terms or used before the first term only.	

A.2.17. Avoid Dangling Phrases

Dangling phrases often are modifiers that do not seem to modify anything. Also, a phrase that is better placed at the beginning of a sentence may be left dangling at the end.

Incorrect	Correct	Note
The clinician selected children for treatment, *taking into consideration the eligibility criteria.*	*Taking into consideration the eligibility criteria,* the clinician selected children for treatment.	
Many undesirable effects of amplification have been eliminated, *with the use of digital hearing aids.*	1. *With the use of digital hearing aids,* many undesirable effects of amplification have been eliminated. 2. Researchers have shown that *digital hearing aids* eliminate many undesirable effects of amplification.	In most cases, fix the dangling phrases by moving them to an earlier position in the sentence.
All children with communicative disorders will be offered treatment, *assuming that we have enough staff available to serve them.*	*Assuming that we have enough staff to serve them,* all children with communicative disorders will be offered treatment.	
I will teach the client self-monitoring skills, *to promote maintenance.*	*To promote maintenance,* I will teach the client self-monitoring skills.	
Children's language problems should not be ignored, *because they can lead to academic failure.*	*Because they can lead to academic failure,* children's language problems should not be ignored.	
Dysarthria is a complex disorder of communication, *affecting most aspects of speech production.*	*Because it affects most aspects of speech production,* dysarthria is a complex disorder of communication.	
Most theories in speech-language pathology are speculative, *they are hard to apply.*	Most theories in speech-language pathology are speculative *and hard to apply.*	

A.2.17. Avoid Dangling Phrases

Incorrect	Write Correctly
I selected assessment procedures, giving much thought to reliability and validity.	
The problems of response maintenance may be handled, using parent training programs.	
Hearing will be tested, with an appropriately calibrated audiometer.	
Ten children will be selected for the study, all with cochlear implants.	
I will teach the client several phonemes this semester, to eliminate his articulation disorder.	
Employers may hesitate to hire persons who stutter, because of the negative attitudes about fluency problems.	
Alzheimer's disease profoundly affects everyone involved, because it changes everything for the patient and the family.	
Hypotheses about language acquisition are hard to verify, they are based on nonexperimental observations.	

A.2.18. Avoid Shifts Within and Between Sentences

Do not shift tense, voice, mood, and number within or between sentences.

Incorrect	Correct	Note
The clinician *was* well trained. She *knows* how to treat a variety of disorders. Nevertheless, she *had* difficulty treating this particular client.	The clinician *was* well trained. She *knew* how to treat a variety of disorders. Nevertheless, she *had* difficulty treating this particular client.	A shift in tense is corrected by maintaining the same past or present tense.
The story *talks* about a man and woman who *fell* in love.	The story *talks* about a man and woman who *fall* in love.	
Van Riper first *developed* an eclectic theory and later a more integrative theory was also *proposed.*	Van Riper first *developed* an eclectic theory and later *proposed* a more integrative theory.	A shift from active to passive voice is corrected by maintaining the active voice.
When *one* is reviewing the literature, *you* find that not many studies have been done on the issue.	When *one* is reviewing the literature, *one* finds that not many studies have been done on the issue.	A shift from second to third person is corrected by maintaining the same pronoun form.
If a *student* studies hard, *you* will impress teachers.	If a *student* studies hard, *he or she* will impress teachers.	A shift from third to second is corrected by maintaining the third person.
If a *client* does not attend at least 90% of the treatment sessions, *they* will not show significant improvement. *Note:* This is an agreement problem as well.	If a *client* does not attend at least 90% of the treatment sessions, *he* or *she* will not show significant improvement.	A shift from singular to plural is corrected by maintaining the singular.
All *hospitals* have *a* physician.	All hospitals have physicians.	A shift from plural to singular is corrected by maintaining the plural.
It is important that an author *buy* a computer and *uses* it regularly.	It is important that an author *buy* a computer and *use* it regularly.	A shift in mood is corrected by maintaining the same imperative mood.

A.2.18. Avoid Shifts Within and Between Sentences

Incorrect	Write Correctly
The client was highly motivated for treatment. Therefore, the progress is good.	
I will first train grammatic morphemes. Later, syntactic features also will be trained.	
When one considers treatment options, you find many alternatives.	
A clinician who does not program maintenance will soon find that they have not completed the treatment.	
The review of the literature shows that this type of experiment has not been conducted. The review also has shown that it is difficult to control all the variables.	
The data suggested that the method was effective. The response rates indicates that maintenance also is enhanced.	
All public schools have a speech-language pathologist.	
If a clinician is exceptional, you are likely to get promoted.	
It is important that a clinician buy recent books and studied them carefully.	
The supervisor observed the client, and then talks to the parent.	

A.2.19. Make Quotations Count

Quotations are borrowed phrases. Good quotations say something effectively and economically. Therefore, do not quote descriptive and ordinary statements.

Descriptive and Ordinary	Rewritten Without Quotations	Note
Not all communicative disorders are related to environmental variables. Research has shown that "many genetic syndromes are associated with communicative disorders" (Brightly, 1993, p. 25).	Not all communicative disorders are related to environmental variables. Research has shown that several genetic syndromes also may be related to communicative disorders (Brightly, 1993).	These quotations do not say anything worth quoting Give reference to specific source of information.
According to Qotme, "aphasia is a common communicative disorder found in the elderly" (1991, p. 9).	Among older people, aphasia is a common communicative disorder.	Common knowledge or general statements do not need a reference.
Quotman stated that "many neurological conditions can be associated with communicative disorders" (1998, p. 589).	Many neurological conditions can be associated with communicative disorders.	
Communicative disorders have a significant effect on the "social, occupational, and personal life of an individual" (Wisdon, 1993, p. 28).	Communicative disorders negatively affect an individual's personal, occupational, and social life (Wisdon, 1993).	
According to Surveyor, "roughly 10% of the population may have a communicative disorder" (1993, p. 18).	It is believed that 10% of the population may have a disorder of communication (Surveyor, 1993).	

A.2.19. Make Quotations Count

Descriptive and Ordinary	Rewrite Without Quotations
According to Linguistron, "many school children have language disorders that go undetected" (1997, p. 50).	
Many researchers "have studied the relation between mild conductive hearing loss and language development" (Otiss, 1998, p. 19).	
During hearing testing, "the clinician should mask the better ear" (Noisley, 1996, p. 567).	
According to Effecton, "some treatment procedures are effective while others are not" (1995, p. 20).	
Brimm has stated that "language acquisition is a complex process" (1989, p. 23).	
"Articulation disorders are common among school-age children" (Soundman, 1998, p. 20).	
"Public schools are an excellent professional setting for speech-language pathologists" (Principal, 1977, p. 1200).	

A.2.20. Do Not Overuse Quotations

Do not use quotations to reduce the amount of your writing. Unless a quote is memorable, paraphrase it and give credit.

Overuse	Judicious Use	Note
The study of language has shown "many rapid changes over the years" (Thomas, 1992, p. 90). In the 1940s "descriptive linguistics dominated the study of language" (TeNiel, 1985, p. 13). According to Thomas (1991), the focus shifted to "transformational generative grammar in the late 1950s and early 1960s" (p. 118). Then again in the 1970s, the focus was shifted to "the essence of language: meaning" (Revolutionary, 1991, p. 50). Soon, however, this approach was abandoned in favor of a "new pragmatic approach" (Bomber, 1989, p. 120).	During the past few decades, the study of language has changed many times. In the 1940s, descriptive linguistics was the main approach to the study of language. Dissatisfied with a purely descriptive study, Chomsky (1957) and others in the late 1950s proposed a new transformational generative grammar approach. In the 1970s, those who disagreed with the purely theoretical grammar approach proposed a new semantic view which focused on "the essence of language: meaning" (Revolutionary, 1991, p. 50). Soon, this, too, was replaced by the newer pragmatic approach (Bomber, 1989).	Overuse of quotations tends to include unremarkable statements as well. Writing littered with ineffective quotes is difficult to read.
Some question whether "apraxia of speech exists in children at all" (Smoothly, 1998, p.27). In the adults, apraxia is "associated with observable signs of neurological disease or trauma" (Brain, 1997, p. 25). Head (1929) has stated that when there is no evidence of neurological involvement, "apraxia of speech in children is a doubtful diagnostic classification" (p. 19).	Some question the existence of apraxia of speech in children. In adults who have apraxia of speech, symptoms of neurological diseases or trauma are documented. Therefore, in the absence of neurological involvement, diagnosis of apraxia in children is questionable (Brain, 1997; Head, 1929; Smoothly, 1998).	

A.2.20. Do Not Overuse Quotations

In rewriting the passages, do not just eliminate the quotation marks. You should rephrase the quotations.

Overuse	Rewrite With Fewer Quotations
Several forms of voice disorders are due to inappropriate behavior. According to Scream, "how you use your voice will determine whether you will have a healthy voice or not" (1992, p. 90). Loud (1987) also stated that "certain occupations pose high risk for voice disorders" (p. 13). Shout said a prudent person avoids "noisy places" (1988, p. 118).	
Either the right or the left ear may be tested first because "the selection is purely arbitrary" (Horton, 1992, p. 32). Research has not shown that it is "better to test one or the other ear first" (McClauey, 1993, p. 67). Most audiologists "begin testing at 1000 Hz, though the order in which the frequencies are tested may not be important" (Soundson, 1991, p. 45). Some audiologists "do not test at 125 Hz at all, while others do" (Southern, 1993, p. 22).	

A.2.21. Do Not Include Islands of Quotations

Instead of standing alone in your writing, quotations should blend smoothly into your expressions.

Incorrect	Correct	Note
Autism is a serious childhood disorder. It starts in early childhood. "Autistic children do not live in the world of their families, but in their own world of distorted fantasy" (Scitzmoore, 1993, p. 10). The disorder affects thought and language. "Autistic children are unable to form emotional bonds with their loved ones" (Sentiment, 1992, p. 15).	Autism is a serious childhood disorder. It starts in early childhood. Autistic children are not in touch with their surroundings as they seem to live "in their own world of distorted fantasy" (Scitzmoore, 1993, p. 10). The disorder affects thought, language, and emotional experience. According to Sentiment (1992), the autistic children are "unable to form emotional bonds with their loved ones" (p. 15).	You quote fewer words when you integrate quotations with your writing. In the correct version, no quotation stands alone. Such phrases as *according to, as stated by, as written by, the author stated that* and so forth help blend a quotation with the main writing.

A.2.22. Do Not Begin a Sentence With a Quotation

Begin sentences with your words. Include quotations within or at the end of your sentence.

Incorrect	Correct
"Cleft palate speech is most readily recognized" (Milton, 1993, p. 20) because of its unique characteristics.	Because of its unique characteristics, "cleft palate speech is most readily recognized" (Milton, 1993, p. 20).
"In recent years, computerized audiometers have been developed to automatically control all aspects of pure tone air- and bone-conduction testing" (Robotson, 1993, p. 98); however, this does not mean that we "do not need audiologists who have a good clinical sense" (Robotson, 1993, p. 99).	In recent years, the administration of hearing tests has been computerized. However, as pointed out by Robotson (1993), we still need audiologists "who have a good clinical sense" (p. 99).

A.2.21. Do Not Include Islands of Quotations

Incorrect	Write Correctly
Multiple misarticulations suggest a need for a phonological process analysis. "A process analysis helps the clinician see order in what might appear to be a collection of random errors" (Godsen, 1992, p. 45). Several methods of phonological analysis are available. "The clinician should select the one that is simple to use and comprehensive in its analysis" (Nixon, 1990, p. 10).	

A.2.22. Do Not Begin a Sentence With a Quotation

Incorrect	Write Correctly
"Audiometers alone, no matter how advanced, will not diagnose hearing impairment" (Torkin, 1993, p. 32). It is the clinician's expert interpretation of results that leads to a clinical diagnosis. "No mechanical device is a substitute for good clinical sense" (Barkin, 1990, p. 551).	
"Specific language disorder often is not associated with an identifiable cause" (Barney, 1992, p. 40). The child may be normal in every respect except for delayed language. "It is hypothesized that specific language delay may have a genetic basis" (Tomokin, 1993, p. 22).	

A.2.23. Use Quotation and Punctuation Marks Correctly

Enclose all direct quotations within two double quotations marks ("and"). Use single quotation marks ('and') to enclose a quotation within a quotation. In most cases, place the punctuation mark **within** the quotation mark. Double check for missing quotation marks at the beginning or the ending of quotations.

Incorrect	Correct	Note
The clinician said, "Good job".	The clinician said, "Good job."	The first two incorrect versions have the punctuation mark outside the quotation marks. The next two have missing quotation marks. In scientific writing, all quotations are referenced.
I will say "wrong", and then mark the incorrect response on the sheet.	I will say "wrong," and then mark the incorrect response on the sheet.	
He said that he was "sorry for what happened.	He said that he was "sorry for what happened."	
According to Soundson, hearing impairment costs billions of dollars to the nation's health care system" (1993, p. 9).	According to Soundson, "hearing impairment costs billions of dollars to the nation's health care system" (1993, p. 9).	

A.2.24. Do Not Overuse Quotation Marks

Do not enclose the following within quotation marks: book and journal titles; technical terms, terms of special emphasis, and linguistic examples. The APA *Manual* requires underlining these; all words underlined in a manuscript will be italicized in print; in term papers, you may italicize them if your instructor approves it.

Incorrect	Correct	Note
"Aphasia: A clinical approach."	Aphasia: A clinical approach. *Aphasia: A clinical approach.*	A book title or a journal name underlined according to the APA *Manual*; italicized otherwise.
"Journal of Audiology"	Journal of Audiology *Journal of Audiology*	
"Dysphonia" means disordered voice.	Dysphonia (or, *Dysphonia*) means disordered voice. **Dysphonia** means disordered voice.	A technical term, defined; underlined, italicized, or in bold-face.
You may not always substitute the conjunction "and" for the ampersand "&."	You may not always substitute the conjunction *and* for the ampersand &.	Linguistic exemplars.

Exception: The titles of articles and papers are neither enclosed within quotation marks nor italicized or underlined. However, titles of theses and dissertations (published or unpublished) are underlined or italicized.

A.2.23. Use Quotation and Punctuation Marks Correctly

Incorrect	Write Correctly
Mrs. Aktsungfoong added that her husband is "stubborn" and "difficult to manage".	
The parents said that their son is "delighted", "very pleased", and "impressed" with the services.	
One expert stated that remediating pragmatic language disorders is the most important treatment target".	

A.2.24. Do Not Overuse Quotation Marks

Incorrect	Write Correctly
"Introduction to Audiology" by Matson	
"Journal of Speech, Language, and Hearing Research"	
"Congenital disorder" is a disorder noticed at the time of birth or soon thereafter.	
The child does not produce the possessive "s" and the present progressive "ing."	

A.2.25. Give References for All Direct Quotations

In scientific writing, all direct quotations should include the following:

- the last name of the author or authors
- the year of publication
- the number of the page or pages on which the quotation is found

Incorrect	Correct	Note
According to Confusius, stuttering is due to "a terrible confusion between who you are and what you want to be.	According to Confucius (1993), stuttering is due to "a terrible confusion between who you are and what you want to be" (p. 37).	The incorrect version includes neither the year of publication nor the page number.
Mixtupton recommended that "children with phonological disorders should be separated from those with a mere articulation disorder" (1993).	Mixtupton recommended that "children with phonological disorders should be separated from those with a mere articulation disorder" (1993, p. 23).	The incorrect version includes the year of publication, but omits the page number.
It has been stated that "chronic and excessively loud speech is detrimental to healthy voice."	It has been stated that "chronic and excessively loud speech is detrimental to healthy voice" (Louden, 1992, p. 10).	The worst of the three, this incorrect version omits the author's name, year of publication, and the page number.
Though stuttering persons may show some excessive anxiety, it is "often associated with speech, and, therefore, there is no evidence for a "trait anxiety" in most stutterers" (Angst, 1991, p. 67).	Though stuttering persons may show some excessive anxiety, it is "often associated with speech, and, therefore, there is no evidence for a 'trait anxiety' in most stutterers" (Angst, 1991, p. 67).	A phrase with double quotation marks within a quotation is enclosed within single quotation marks.
Although found in all societies, "the incidence of cleft palate varies across different racial groups, suggesting the importance of genetic factors in its etiology" (Geneson, 1990, pp. 10–11).	Although found in all societies, "the incidence of cleft palate varies across different racial groups, suggesting the importance of genetic factors in its etiology" (Geneson, 1990, pp. 10–11).	The correct version shows the page on which the quotation begins and the page on which it ends. p. for one page. pp. for two or more pages. Both in lower case.

Note: There are different methods of placing the name, the year, and the page number. The period is placed only after the parenthetical closure, not before or after the quotation marks.

A.2.25. Give References for All Direct Quotations

Invent the information that is necessary to write correctly.

Incorrect	Write Correctly
According to Loveson, language delay is due to "many factors but none can be directly traced to lack of parental love for the child."	
Boontenthorpe has written that "adults who have strokes and aphasia show remarkable spontaneous recovery within three to six months of onset" (1993).	
It has been stated that "a single, loud scream can damage the vocal cords."	
A neglected cause of hearing impairment is "the types of food we eat; it is possible that "pesticide-laced grains and fruits" are a source of cochlear damage in some cases" (Peston, 1991, p. 67).	
Recent developments in cochlear implants have "made it possible for many deaf children to begin their aural rehabilitation early in life" (Coplant, 1990, p. 15–16).	

A.2.26. Reproduce Quotations Exactly

Make quotations identical to the original in words, spelling, and punctuation. Reproduce errors as they are in the original with the insertion of the word [*sic*], italicized (or underlined), and placed within brackets.

A Quotation With an Error in It	Note
Numbasa's description of language as a mental phenomenon "that can be studied only by some powerfil [*sic*] intuitive procedures" was especially appealing to clinicians who had based their treatment procedures on intuition.	In the quotation, the italicized word [*sic*] suggests that in the original, the word *powerful* is misspelled.

A.2.27. Integrate Quotations of Less Than 40 Words With the Text

Incorrect (Unintegrated)	Correct	Note
Numbasa defined language as: "A cognitive ability to synthesize and symbolize mental experience and to represent this experience in patterns of sounds, words, and sentences following linguistic rules that are innately given" (1971, p. 95)	Numbasa defined language as "a cognitive ability to synthesize and symbolize mental experience and to represent this experience in patterns of sounds, words, and sentences following linguistic rules that are innately given" (1971, p. 95).	Only quotations of 40 words or more are set off from the rest of the text. See A.2.28.

A.2.28. *Block* Quotations When They Have 40 or More Words

- A quotation set apart from the text is a block quotation.
- Type quotations of 40 words or more as block quotations.
- Type the entire quotation indented five spaces from the left margin.
- Indent the first line of the second (and subsequent) paragraphs five more spaces.
- Do not use quotation marks.
- However, place within double quotation marks a quotation within a block quotation.
- After the quotation, type the page number of the quotation within parentheses.
- Do not type a period after the closing parenthesis.

A.2.26. Reproduce Quotations Exactly

Quotation With an Error in It	Quote It Appropriately
Dinson (1987) said that "language is not to be confused with what people say, because language is a metal tool of imagination" (p. 40).	

A.2.27. Integrate Quotations of Less Than 40 Words With the Text

Incorrectly Arranged Quotation	Integrate the Quote With Text
Galle (1993) stated that: Every child who learns to speak his or her language is a scientist who tests alternative hypotheses about the nature of language. The spoken language the child hears is the data for hypothesis testing. (p. 23) This statement made a profound impact on the study of language and its natural acquisition. This statement also is popular with many clinicians.	*Hint:* Write a single paragraph containing the quotation.

Block Quotations (continued)

Block Quotation	Note
In his powerful explanation of language intervention, Mumbasa (1991) has stated the following:	
Language intervention is a process of unleashing powerful but painfully hidden but unconsciously active communicative potential. The goals of language intervention include transcendental self-actualization, cognitive reorganization, and reconstruction of perceptual-emotive reality.	Indent the first line of the block quotation by five spaces from the left margin. Do not use quotation marks. Double-space the quotation as you would the text; do not give extra space before or after a block quotation.
The process of language intervention is mysterious. A successful clinician has an innate ability to solve this mystery. (p. 19)	Indent the second paragraph of the quotation by five *more* spaces. Give one space before the first parenthesis enclosing the page number. Do not type a period after the closing parenthesis.
Mumbasa's explanation is now a basis for many language treatment programs. Clinicians who despise tiresome objectivity in language treatment have gladly adopted this view.	Begin your text with a new paragraph.

A.2.28. *Block* Quotations When They Have 40 or More Words

Quotation of More Than 40 Words	Arrange It Properly
Confidon (1992) has stated that "the root cause of stuttering is lack of a shining self-image. That fluent speech is a function of self-image that throws bright light into the eyes of the listener is well established. Therefore, to make stuttering persons speak fluently, we must find ways of polishing their self-image so it begins to shine again" (pp. 35–36). All clinicians should consider this powerful explanation of stuttering in planning treatment for their clients. Treatment based on this explanation will undoubtedly solve the nagging problem of maintenance of fluency.	

A.2.29. Show Correctly the Changes in Quotations

- When you omit words from a sentence within a quotation, insert three ellipsis marks with a space before and after each mark (e.g., mark . . .).
- When you omit words between sentences, insert four ellipsis marks; the first of these four is a period, hence no space before it; the three other marks are separated by a space; there is a space after the third mark (e.g., mark. . . .).
- Do not insert ellipsis marks at the beginning and end of a quotation even when it begins or ends in midsentence.
- If you insert words into a quotation, enclose them within brackets.
- Underline (as per the APA *Manual*) or italicize (if acceptable in a term paper) the words you emphasize that were not emphasized in the original.
- Next to the underlined or italicized word, type the words [italics added] within brackets.

Changed Quotation	Note
Bluff has stated that "stuttering cannot be measured by . . . merely counting dysfluencies. Stuttering and dysfluencies are not to be confused. . . . It [stuttering] is more than *mere dysfluencies*" [italics added] (1993, p. 58).	Omitted words within a sentence indicated: *by . . . merely* Omitted words between sentences indicated: *confused. . . . It* (a period, three dots, and two spaces) Inserted word bracketed: *It* [stuttering] *is*

A.2.29. Show Correctly the Changes in Quotations

Changed Quotation	Rewrite Correctly
Snuff has stated that "Voice disorders are not only a product of various medical pathologies (words omitted) but also a product of certain life styles. Therefore, clinicians should take a careful and detailed history of the client (words omitted at the end of the sentence). Information obtained through history is invaluable in planning treatment for voice clients (the last three words added). They (the clinicians: added words) should not hesitate to probe the client's life style" (italics not in the original) (1990, p. 50).	

A.2.30. Use Latin Abbreviations Only in Parenthetical Constructions

In nonparenthetical written sentences, use their English equivalents; do not use Latin abbreviations in conversational speech.

Abbreviation	English Equivalent
etc.	and so forth
e.g.,	for example
i.e.,	that is
viz.,	namely
cf.	compare
vs.	versus, against

Exceptions:

1. Use the abbreviation v. for versus when referring to court cases: The historic Brown v. Board of Education ruling has been upheld.
2. Use the Latin abbreviation et al., which means "and others" in parenthetical and nonparenthetical writing. See B.3.32 for examples.

Incorrect	Correct
Pictures, objects, line drawings, etc. will be used as stimuli.	Pictures, objects, line drawings, and so forth will be used as stimuli.
Various reinforcers, e.g., tokens, stickers, and points, will be used as reinforcers.	Various reinforcers, for example, tokens, stickers, and points, will be used as reinforcers.
The basic continuous reinforcement schedule, i.e., the fixed ratio 1 (FR1), may be used.	The basic continuous reinforcement schedule, that is, the fixed ratio 1(FR1), may be used.
Certain variables, *viz.*, motivation, severity of the disorder, and intelligence are known to influence the treatment outcome.	Certain variables, namely, motivation, severity of the disorder, and intelligence are known to influence the treatment outcome.
Nativism vs. empiricism is a historical topic of discussion.	Nativism versus empiricism is a historical topic of discussion.

A.2.30. Use Latin Abbreviations Only in Parenthetical Constructions

Take note of an exception, however.

Incorrect	Write Correctly
Interjections, prolongations, repetitions, etc. are among the types of dysfluencies.	
Certain types of newer hearing aids, e.g., the digital aids, can reduce background noise.	
Neural hearing loss, i.e., the type of loss with nerve damage, is difficult to treat surgically.	
Many variables, viz., heredity, environmental toxicity, and maternal alcoholism can cause mental retardation.	
Behaviorism vs. cognitivism is a good topic for debate.	
The Brown versus the Board of Education ruling forced racial integration in public schools.	

A.2.31. Avoid Euphemism

Euphemistic expressions disguise negative meanings. Such expressions falsely suggest neutral or positive meanings. Euphemistic writing can be dishonest.

Euphemistic	Direct
Because of poor progress, the family will be *counseled out* of our services.	1. Because of poor progress, the family will be dismissed from our services. 2. Because of poor progress, we recommended to the family that our services be discontinued.
The client is *communicatively challenged.*	1. The client has a communicative disorder. 2. The client has an articulation problem.
The child comes from an *economically deprived* background.	The child comes from a poor family.
The child is *mentally other-abled.*	The child is mentally retarded.
He is a *residentially challenged* person.	He is a homeless person.

A.2.32. Avoid Jargon

Jargon is a technical or specialized term; sometimes it is unavoidable.

Do not overuse jargon.

When necessary, describe what jargon means in everyday language.

When you write to persons without technical knowledge, describe everything in nontechnical terms.

When writing to technical audiences, retain the technical terms.

Jargon	Plain
The child's *linguistic competence* is limited.	The child's *language* is limited.
Use an *FR2 schedule* to reinforce correct responses at home.	Reinforce *every other correct response* at home.
In using your hearing aid, you should learn to control the *intensity of the signal.*	In using your hearing aid, you should learn to control the *volume.*
The child's *MLU* is limited.	The child speaks in *short phrases or sentences.*
The woman has *anomia.*	The woman has naming difficulties.

A.2.31. Avoid Euphemism

Euphemistic	Write More Directly
The student was counseled out of the major.	
The child comes from an underprivileged family.	
The man is physically challenged.	
Today, the garbologist did not collect the trash.	
I bought a previously owned car.	
We will give you another opportunity to take the comprehensive examination.	

A.2.32. Avoid Jargon

Jargon	Write in Plain Language
The boy has a severe problem in correctly positioning his articulators.	
The child has telegraphic speech.	
The woman has aphonia.	
Your child has a final consonant deletion process.	

A.2.33. Use the Terms Ending With *-ology* (and Some With *-ics*) Correctly

A few terms that end with *-ology* are frequently misused even in scholarly and clinical writing. *-Ology* is a study of something or a branch of learning; *-ics* in certain words also is a suffix that means the study of something; use terms that end with these suffixes only to refer to a branch of learning or a study of something.

Incorrect	Correct	Note
The child had a disordered morphology.	The child's morphologic productions were impaired. The child does not produce certain morphologic features.	*Disordered morphology* means chaotic study of morphologic aspects of language!
His morphology needs attention.	His morphological skills need attention.	Does his study of morphologic aspects of language need attention?
The disordered phonology was a major clinical concern.	The phonologic disorder was a major concern.	Is the study of phonologic aspects of language disordered?
She described the child's phonology.	She described the child's phonological performance.	Did the child produce a branch of learning called phonology?
His semantics is impaired.	His understanding of meaning (semantic features) is impaired. His productions suggest impaired semantic skills.	Semantics is the study of meaning in language; it cannot be impaired.
The training should concentrate on her semantics.	The training should concentrate on her semantic features.	Should the training concentrate on her study of meaning?
The client's pragmatics needs help.	The client's pragmatic skills need help (treatment).	Does the client's study of use of language need help?
The disordered pragmatics requires advanced training.	The disordered pragmatic features require advanced training.	Does the study of pragmatic aspects of language require advanced training?
Because of his cancer, his physiology is disordered.	Because of his cancer, his physiological system is upset.	These less common mistakes point out the inappropriateness of *disordered phonology* and *impaired morphology.*
A brain tumor implies disordered neurology.	A brain tumor implies a neurological disorder (disease).	

A.2.33. Use the Terms Ending With *-ology* (and Some With *-ics*) Correctly

Incorrect	Write Correctly
The client has a disturbed morphology.	
The child's morphology should be targeted for treatment.	
The assessment results show that the child's phonology is disordered.	
A good description of a client's phonology is essential before starting phonologic treatment.	
Her semantics is difficult to analyze.	
Semantics was one of the treatment goals.	
His use of pragmatics is questionable.	
Her pragmatics should be a treatment target.	
Her biology is impaired.	
His psychology is disturbed.	

A.2.34. Avoid Clichés

Clichés are overused and dull expressions; they include most idioms. Replace clichés and idioms with more appropriate words.

Cliché	Simple and Direct	Note
We do not have many *tried-and-true* treatment techniques.	We do not have many proven treatment techniques.	The word *proven* is more acceptable for this kind of writing.
Though he recently had a stroke, the patient was *fit as a fiddle*.	Though he recently had a stroke, the patient was in good health.	An everyday term is more appropriate than the cliché.
Treating patients with laryngectomy is not her *cup of tea*.	1. She does not enjoy treating patients with laryngectomy. 2. She does not know how to treat patients with laryngectomy.	Some clichés mask multiple meanings.
In *this day and age*, the clinician needs to have computer skills.	The clinician now needs to have computer skills.	

A.2.35. Avoid Colloquial or Informal Expressions

The rule applies to scientific and professional writing.

Informal	Formal	Note
If the client *can't* imitate, I will use the shaping method.	If the client *cannot* imitate, I will use the shaping method.	Avoid informal contractions.
Continuous reinforcement *won't* be used.	Continuous reinforcement *will not* be used.	
The researcher *felt* that the procedure was effective.	The researcher *thought* that the procedure was effective.	Avoid such subjective terms as *felt* unless the reference is to feelings.
The clinician should *get across* the idea that maintenance treatment is important.	The clinician should *point out* that maintenance treatment is important.	Colloquial expressions
The clinician *came up* with a dysphagia assessment procedure.	The clinician *developed* a dysphagia assessment procedure.	

A.2.34. Avoid Clichés

Cliché	Write in Simple and Direct Words
The child is bored to tears with therapy.	
The initial progress gave the client a shot in the arm.	
The child who stutters is sick and tired of teasing from her friends.	
In promoting maintenance, I will leave no stone unturned.	
My treatment plan was off the track.	

A.2.35. Avoid Colloquial or Informal Expressions

Informal	Formal
The client just wouldn't imitate the modeled stimulus.	
The clinician hadn't prepared the stimulus materials.	
I feel that the client's hoarseness of voice is due to vocal nodules.	
In counseling the parents of a child with a hearing loss, you should get across the idea that the early intervention is important.	
The clinician cooked-up a novel method of evoking the /r/.	

A.3. COMMONLY MISUSED WORDS AND PHRASES

Use the following words or phrases correctly. Know the differential meaning of the words that often are confused.

A.3.1. Affect and Effect

Generally, use *affect* as a verb and *effect* as a noun. **Exceptions:** Use *effect* (or the term to *effect*) always as a verb or verb phrase when the meaning is *to cause a change* or *create an effect*; (2) use *affect* as a noun when it refers to an emotional state (e.g., *When he lost the bet, his affect changed*).

Incorrect	Correct
Many researchers have studied the masking noise *affect* on stuttering.	Many researchers have studied the masking noise *effect* on stuttering.
She studied the treatment *affects*.	She studied the treatment *effects*.
The treatment *effected* the behavior.	The treatment *affected* the behavior.
How did the variable *effect* the outcome?	How did the variable *affect* the outcome?
The clinician's goal is to *affect* changes in the client's communicative behaviors.	The clinician's goal is to *effect* changes in the client's communicative behaviors.
The clinician could not *affect* changes in the patient's naming skills.	The clinician could not *effect* changes in the patient's naming skills.

A.3.2. Alternate and Alternative

Alternate means different events occurring or succeeding by turns; to alternate is to shift from one to the other. *Alternative* suggests a choice between two possibilities.

Incorrect	Correct	Note
We will use the two *alternative* treatments to see if one is more effective than the other.	We will *alternate* the two treatments to see if one is better than the other.	Clinician shifts from one treatment to the other; both are offered in different sessions.
The appliance uses *alternative* current	The appliance uses *alternating* current	Current reverses its direction at regular intervals.
I will take the *alternative* route.	I will take the *alternate* route.	The person took the other route; it is one or the other.
The only *alternate* to treatment is continued stuttering.	The only *alternative* to treatment is continued stuttering.	The statement says there is only one choice.

A.3. COMMONLY MISUSED WORDS AND PHRASES

A.3.1. Affect and Effect

Incorrect	Write Correctly
The affect of environmental deprivation on language acquisition is significant.	
This study on the affect of aphasia treatment was poorly designed.	
Modeling effected the target response.	
How does the parental dysfluency rate effect the child's stuttering?	
To effect changes in clients' behaviors, the clinician needs strong treatment programs.	
In spite of her excellent efforts, the clinician could not affect changes in the patient's cognitive skills.	

A.3.2. Alternate and Alternative

Incorrect	Write Correctly
It leaves me with no alternate.	
You can alternative the two probe procedures.	
We will alternatively use auditory comprehension and speech production to see which one is more effective.	
The alternate to college education is a low paying job.	

A.3.3. Allusion and Illusion

Use *illusion* to refer to an unreal image and *allusion* to suggest an indirect reference.

Incorrect	Correct
She made an *illusion* to the new theory of voice production.	She made an *allusion* to the new theory of voice production.
The ghost he thought he saw was merely an *allusion*.	The ghost he thought he saw was merely an *illusion*.

A.3.4. And/Or

Do not write *and/or*. Rewrite the sentence.

Incorrect	Correct
Pictures *and/or* objects will be used to evoke the target behaviors.	Pictures, objects, *or both* will be used to evoke the target behaviors.
Speech-language pathologists *and/or* psychologists may assess patients with aphasia.	Speech-language pathologists, psychologists, *or both* may assess patients with aphasia.

A.3.5. Farther and Further

Use *farther* to refer to distance. Use *further* to refer to time or quantity.

Incorrect	Correct
She walked *further* than any person did.	She walked *farther* than any person.
I sent the parents a *farther* notice of an IEP meeting.	I sent the parents a *further* notice of an IEP meeting.
Farthermore, the client was often late.	*Furthermore*, the client was often late.

A.3.3. Allusion and Illusion

Incorrect	Write Correctly
He made an illusion to an emerging trend in the treatment of dysarthria.	
The treatment effects reported in the study were merely an allusion.	

A.3.4. And/Or

Incorrect	Write Correctly
The father and/or the mother of the client will be trained in response maintenance.	
Language disorders and/or phonological disorders may coexist with stuttering.	

A.3.5. Farther and Further

Incorrect	Write Correctly
New York is further than you think.	
After establishing the target behaviors, the clinician should do farther work on maintenance.	
I will study the subject farther.	

A.3.6. Incidence and Prevalence

Incidence refers to the future occurrence of an event in a population. *(How many normally speaking children will begin to stutter?)*

Prevalence refers to the current existence; you take a head count. *(How many children in the school district have a hearing impairment?)*

Note that the word *incidence* often is misused; prevalence is more appropriate in such cases.

Incorrect	Correct	Note
The *incidence* of stuttering in the population of the United States is about 2 million.	The *incidence* of stuttering in the population of the United States is about 1%.	Incidence of stuttering refers to the number of people who are expected to stutter.
The *prevalence* of hearing impairment is about 10%.	The *prevalence* of 2,000 children with hearing impairment requires additional services. The *incidence* of hearing impairment is about 10%.	Prevalence refers to the total number of persons who already have a characteristic or a disorder.

A.3.7. Inter- and Intra-

Inter- means *between or among. Intra-* means *within.*

Incorrect	Correct	Note
The *intraobserver* reliability index is based on the observation of two graduate students.	*Intraobserver* reliability is based on two observations of the experimenter.	To determine *intraobserver* reliability, the same person should repeat observations.
The *interobserver* reliability index is based on the experimenter's two observations.	The *interobserver* reliability index is based on the observations of two experts.	Two determine *interobserver* reliability, two or more persons should observe the same event.
I will take an *intrastate* highway to cross the state boundary.	I will take an *interstate* highway to cross the state boundary.	An interstate highway runs across states.
Motivation is an *interpersonal* variable.	Motivation is an *intrapersonal* variable.	Motivation is a within-person factor.

A.3.6. Incidence and Prevalence

Incorrect	Write Correctly
The incidence of strokes in the country is about 500,000.	
The prevalence of language disorders in the school-age children in the city is 10%.	

A.3.7. Inter- and Intra-

Incorrect	Correct
I will establish the intraobserver reliability by correlating my observations with those of another observer.	
The experimenter established an interobserver reliability index by correlating two of her observations.	
Minimally two observers are needed to calculate an intraobserver reliability index.	
The same observer has to make minimally two observations to calculate an interobserver reliability index.	

A.3.8. Latter and Later

Latter means the second of the two things just mentioned; contrasts with *former*, which means the first of the two things just mentioned.

Later has a specific reference to time: it refers to something done after another activity or time period.

Incorrect	Correct	Note
In the beginning I will work on establishment, *latter* I will work on maintenance.	In the beginning, I will teach the target behaviors, *later* I will train parents to promote maintenance.	Your work on maintenance comes later in time.
Your training criterion may be 80% or 90% correct; the *later* requires more training.	Your training criterion may be 80% or 90% correct; the *latter* requires more training.	The latter refers to the second of the two criteria mentioned (90%). The term helps avoid repetition of an element.

A.3.9. Secondly and Thirdly

Avoid this usage. Write: *First, Second, Third*, and so forth.

Not Preferred	Preferred	Note
First, I will assess the client. *Secondly*, I will select the target behaviors. *Thirdly*, I will prepare the stimulus materials.	First, I will assess the client. *Second*, I will select the target behaviors. *Third*, I will prepare the stimulus materials.	Some write *firstly*, but it is worse than *secondly* and *thirdly*.

A.3.10. Since and Because

The word *since* often is misused.

Use *since* to suggest a temporal (time) sequence, as in *Since the introduction of in-the-ear hearing aids, social acceptability of hearing aid usage has increased.*

Use *because* to suggest causation, as in *Because the man stuttered, he felt self-conscious.*

Incorrect	Correct	Note
Since the stimulus pictures are ambiguous, the responses are not certain.	*Because* the stimulus pictures are ambiguous, the responses are not certain.	Uncertain responses are due to ambiguous pictures.

A.3.8. Later and Latter

Incorrect	Correct
I am busy now; will do it latter.	
First, I will teach the target behaviors; latter I will probe for generalized productions.	
Clinicians offer direct treatment to children and counseling to parents; the later requires additional clinical skills.	
I had an introductory text and an advanced text for the course. I liked the former, but hated the later.	

A.3.9. Secondly and Thirdly

Not Preferred	Preferred
First, I will instruct the client on what he or she should do. Secondly, I will place the headphones on the client. Thirdly, I will begin hearing testing.	

A.3.10. Since and Because

Incorrect	Write Correctly
Since the auditory discrimination procedure was not effective, I shifted to production training.	
Since the child is not cooperative, automatic audiologic assessment procedures are necessary.	

A.3.11. Elicit and Evoke

In speech-language pathology, the word *elicit* is widely used to describe procedures that stimulate communicative behaviors. A more accurate word, however, is *evoke*. A stimulus evokes a voluntary response and *elicits* a reflexive response. For example, a tap on the knee *elicits* the knee-jerk reflex, whereas a picture and a question *evoke* the naming response from a patient with aphasia.

Less Accurate	More Accurate	Note
I will *elicit* a language sample from the child with the help of toys.	I will *evoke* a language sample from the child.	Technically, reflexive responses are *elicited* and voluntary responses are *evoked*. Speech and language are not reflexive responses.
I will *evoke* dilation of the pupil by a flash of light.	I will *elicit* dilatioxn of the pupil.	
Pavlov *evoked* the salivary reflex by placing meat powder in the dog's mouth.	Pavlov *elicited* the salivary reflex by placing meat powder in the dog's mouth.	
By reinforcing them, Skinner *elicited* and increased the bar pressing responses in rats.	By reinforcing them, Skinner *evoked* and increased the bar pressing responses in rats.	

A.3.12. Elicit and Illicit

Because of an especially troublesome confusion, some students try to *illicit target responses*. The phrase makes no sense because *illicit* is not even a verb—it is an adjective—but a supervisor with no sense of humor may pull out handcuffs!

Incorrect	Correct	Note
Pictures will be used to *illicit* the phoneme.	Pictures will be used to *evoke* the phoneme.	The less accurate *elicit* is preferable to the illegal *illicit*.
I will teach the mother to *illicit* the target behaviors at home.	I will teach the mother to *evoke* the target behaviors at home.	

A.3.11. Elicit and Evoke

Less Accurate	Write More Accurately
Pavlov evoked the salivary reflex.	
Skinner elicited the bar press response.	
There are many procedures to elicit the production of /s/.	
I will evoke the psychogalvanic reflex.	
I know a few methods of evoking the swallow reflex.	

A.3.12. Elicit and Illicit

Incorrect	Write Correctly
She illicited single-word responses form her client.	
I will demonstrate in front of a mirror to illicit /k/.	
I will use pictures to illicit naming responses from my patient with aphasia.	

Note: There is no such word as *illicited*.

A.3.13. Compare to and Compare with

To compare is to point out similarities *and* differences between two things. The term *compare to* is used to describe similarities; the term *compare with* is used to describe differences and similarities, but mostly differences.

Incorrect	Correct	Note
The brain is *compared with* a computer because the two seem to perform similar functions.	The brain is *compared to* a computer because the two seem to perform similar functions.	The authors mean to describe similarity between the brain and the computer in the first example and that between language acquisition and hypothesis testing in the second example; hence, *compared to*.
Children's language acquisition is *compared with* the scientific process of hypothesis testing.	Children's language acquisition is *compared to* the scientific process of hypothese testing.	
You should *compare* the revised version of the paper *to* its original to see how much it has changed.	You should *compare* the revised version of the paper *with* its original to see how much it hs changed.	The emphasis is on the difference between the two versions or courses at two levels, although some similarities also may be noted; hence, *compare with*.
When you *compare* graduate seminars *to* the undergraduate courses, you will be amazed by the differences.	When you *compare* graduate seminars *with* undergraduate courses, you will be amazed by the differences.	

A.3.14. Compare and Contrast

To *contrast* two things is to point out differences between them. Because *compare* can be used to point out similarities and differences between objects (see A.3.13), the phrase *compare and contrast* is redundant.

Incorrect	Correct	Note
Because they hardly share any similarities, the instructor *compared* the nativist theory *to* the behavioral theory of language.	Because they hardly share any similarities, the instructor *contrasted* the nativist theory *with* the behavioral theory . of language	The instructor described differences, not similarities; hence, *contrasted*
The fluency shaping procedures may be *compared* with stutter-more-fluently approaches for their opposing strategies.	The fluency shaping procedures may be *contrasted with* stutter-more-fluently approaches for their opposing strategies.	Describing opposing strategies; hence, *contrasted*

A.3.13. Compare to and Compare with

Incorrect	Write Correctly
The human body is compared with a machine because both have a structure capable of certain functions.	
When stuttering treatment is compared with cluttering treatment, more similarities than differences are evident.	
If you compare the phonological approach to the distinctive feature approach, you will see how different they are in suggesting treatment strategies for articulation disorders.	
When you compare academic courses with clinical practicum, you will see many differences.	

A.3.14. Compare and Contrast

Incorrect	Write Correctly
When compared to the single-phoneme approach, the multiple phoneme approach appears vastly different.	
The gray winter, compared to colorful spring, has a different effect on my mood.	
The single phoneme approach may be compared with multiple phoneme approach for their distinctively different approaches.	

A.3.15. Effect and Impact

Effect is a classic term in scientific writing used to describe the change one variable causes in another. There is no point in substituting *effect* with *impact*, a vogue word whose original meaning is *striking of one body against the other*; it also means *to pack firmly*, as in the expression *the audiologist found impacted wax in the client's ear*. Many critics who once despised the term impact when used to suggest *effect* have become resigned to its ever-escalating force (impact!) of popularity.

Inaccurate	Accurate	Note
Modeling has an *impact* on the client's productions.	Modeling has an *effect* on the client's productions.	Modeling does not strike or firmly pack the client's productions.
This treatment is known to have an *impact*.	This treatment is known to have an *effect*.	The traditional word does fine.

A.3.16. Focus and Analysis (Study)

Focus is another vogue word whose popularity is ever escalating. People do not pay attention to anything any more; they just *focus*. In scientific writing, the words *focus* and *focusing* distract the scientist from using more precise terms, including *study* or *analysis*.

Vague	More Precise	Note
She *focused* on the principles of aerobic dancing.	In her lecture, she *concentrated* on the principles of aerobic dancing.	The inaccurate statement does not say what the lecturer did.
To prevent heart diseases, scientists are *focusing* on people's dietary habits.	To find a cure for heart diseases, scientists are *studying* people's dietary habits.	Just focusing on a problem may not help solve it.
In solving the crime problem, investigators have *focused* on family dynamics.	In solving the crime problem, investigators have *analyzed* family dynamics.	

A.3.15. Effect and Impact

Inaccurate	Accurate
Slow rate of speech has a profound impact on stuttering.	
Several investigators have analyzed the impact of noise on speech.	
The impact of treatment was negligible.	

A.3.16. Focus and Analysis (Study)

Vague	Write More Precisely
Because I am getting poor grades, I need to focus on my study skills.	
The instructor focused on some difficult theories.	
The researchers now focus on the genetic bases of hearing impairment.	

A.3.17. There and Their

Use *there* to suggest location and *their* to suggest group possession.

Incorrect	Correct	Note
This is *there* house.	This is *their* house	A common mistake.
Their is the book you wanted.	*There is* the book you wanted,	
Was *their* supposed to be a party tonight?	Was *there* supposed to be a party tonight?	
How is *there* health?	How is *their* health?	

A.3.18. Accept and Except

The two do not share meaning, but the confusion between the two may be due to phonetic similarity. *Accept* means to receive something offered; *except* means with the exclusion of (something or someone). Erroneous substitution of *except* for *accept* is a common mistake.

Incorrect	Correct	Note
I *except* your kind offer.	I *accept* your kind offer.	The incorrect expressions do not make sense.
She *excepted* our gift.	She graciously *accepted* our gift.	
I was the only one *accepted* from the regulation.	I was the only one *excepted* from the regulation	
All were admitted into the bar, *accept* me.	All were admitted into the bar, *except* me.	
I will *except* all conditions *accept* the first.	I will *accept* all conditions *except* the first.	The incorrect expressions may be interpreted to mean the opposite of what is intended.
Scientists have *excepted* most of these hypotheses, *accept* perhaps the last two.	Scientists have *accepted* most of these hypotheses, except perhaps the last two.	

A.3.17. There and Their

Incorrect	Write Correctly
That was once there haunt.	
Their is what you need.	
I though their was going to be a quiz today.	
How is there new baby?	

A.3.18. Accept and Except

Incorrect	Write More Precisely
I am pleased to except your job offer.	
He did not except our offer of assistance.	
Everyone got in, accept John.	
The faculty excepted all applicants, accept one.	
Scientists have excepted these theories, accept perhaps the first.	

A.3.19. Baseline and Baserate

Use *baseline* only as a noun. Use *baserate* as a verb or as a noun. Note that the word *baserate* (or *baseline*) is a single word; they are not written as *base rate* or *base line*.

Incorrect	Correct	Note
Before starting treatment, the clinician should *baseline* target behaviors.	Before starting treatment, the clinician should establish *baselines* of target behaviors.	*Baselines* incorrectly used as a verb and correctly used as a noun.
I *baselined* the target responses.	I will establish *baselines* of target responses.	
I *will baseline* phoneme productions.	I will *baserate* phoneme productions. I will measure the *baserate* of phoneme productions.	*Baseline* incorrectly used as a verb and correctly substituted with *baserate*. *Baserate* correctly used as a verb.

A.3.20. Proof and Support

In scientific writing, use the word *proof* or *proved* sparingly. Scientists rarely prove a hypothesis; they only support it with evidence or reject it (by failing to support it). The same comments apply to *disprove*, as the examples show.

Less Accurate	More Accurate	Note
My data *prove* that there is a gene for transformational generative grammar.	My data *support* the hypothesis that there is a gene for transformational generative grammar.	Beside *support*, several other words are good substitutes for *proof*.
These observations *prove* that the treatment was effective.	These observations *suggest* that the treatment was effective.	
Johnson *proved* that the Native Americans do not stutter.	Johnson *claimed* that the Native Americans do not stutter.	The word *claimed* suggests that the author is skeptic of the hypothesis.
More recent studies have *disproved* Johnson's claim.	More recent studies have *contradicted* Johnson's claim.	

A.3.19. Baseline and Baserate

Incorrect	Write Correctly
All target behaviors should be baselined before starting treatment.	
I first baselined the turn taking in conversation.	
I will baseline morphologic productions.	1. Correct noun form: 2. Correct verb form

A.3.20. Proof and Support

Less Accurate	Write Accurate
The linguists have proved that there is an innate language acquisition device.	
My data prove that the hypothesis is invalid.	
Chimpsky proved that all children are born with universal grammar.	
Recent research disproves Chimpsky's claim.	

Note to Student Writers

Examples on the previous pages sample only a small number of commonly misused words and phrases. Use this page to write down additional examples of such words and phrases. Practice correct usage of those words and phrases.

Misused Words	Correct Usage

Note: The APA *Manual* has a few additional examples; many books on writing contain sections on word usage.

PART B

SCIENTIFIC WRITING

B.I. PRINCIPLES OF SCIENTIFIC WRITING

Printed Notes	Class Notes

Scientific writing is:

- related to data, research, or theory
- direct
- precise
- objective
- organized according to an accepted format.

Scientific papers have somewhat rigid formats. Different scientific journals have their specific formats.

Journals the American Speech-Language-Hearing Association (ASHA) publishes use a format that is based on the *Publication Manual of the American Psychological Association* (APA *Manual*, 4th edition).

However, please take note that ASHA journals do not strictly follow the APA format. In heading styles and reference citations, for example, the ASHA journals use a different style than the one recommended by the APA *Manual*.

All writing is designed for an audience. In addition, scientific and professional writing also is designed for an agency or a source of publication or agency. For example, a research paper may be designed according to the format presecribed by a journal to which it is submitted. A grant proposal, on the other hand, may be designed according to the guidelines of a government agency or a private foundation.

Undergraduate and graduate students write term papers. Advanced graduate students may write research papers, theses, and dissertations. In completing

Printed Notes	Class Notes

their writing projects, students should follow a prescribed format. The instructor of a course, the graduate school, or a departmental policy may dictate the format.

Students should find out the accepted or prescribed format and write accoringly. Throughout this part on scientific writing, the APA style is used for illustration.

There always are reasons to deviate from a particular style. You should ascertain from your instructor the acceptable deviations from the prescribed style. Potential or recommended deviations from the APA *Manual* guidelines are specified in this section.

Please note that a book, such is this one, does not fully conform to the APA style in its headings, paragraph indentations, margins, the use of italics and underlining, and so forth. General design features that are appropriate for an article or a term paper may not be appropriate for a book. Each publishing company uses its own style in designing books. For esthetic reasons, headings, paragraph styles, and so forth often are uniquely designed for each book. Therefore, students should not look at book designs, including the design of this book, to understand the APA style.

An important skill to acquire is *writing without bias*. Scientific writing should be free from racial, cultural, ethnic, social, economic, and gender-related biases. Negative connotations about disabilities, unless such connotations are a matter of scientific study, also should be avoided.

Scientific writing avoids stereotypic language about sexes, individuals, and ethnic groups. Scientific writing makes reference

Printed Notes	Class Notes

to ethnic, racial, and other cultural factors only when:

- those factors themselves are the subject of a study
- the knowledge of such factors is necessary to understand the results of a study or issues on hand

Necessary references to gender, culture, ethnicity, and race are made in:

- nonevaluative and nonoffensive language
- terms that groups use to refer to themselves

Gender bias is the most frequent problem. Implied or direct negative reference to disabilities also is a frequent problem.

Note that biases are not just a problem in scientific writing. They are a problem in:

- all writing
- conversational speech
- media reports

Your speech and writing should be free from biases. The APA *Manual* has guidelines on writing without racial, gender-related, and other kinds of biases. Study those guidelines. On the following pages, you will find examples of and exercises for writing without bias.

B.2.1. Write Without Gender Bias

Terms That Suggest Bias	Appropriate Use	Note
Man	Use only when you refer to a male person	
Mankind	*humankind, humans, people*	
he his (other male referents)	*he or she* [but not *he/she*, nor *(s)he*] *his* or *her*	Of course, the male referents are fine if the reference is restricted to male persons.
Animals share only a part of *man's* capacity for communication.	Animals share only a part of *humans'* capacity for communication.	
The recent scientific achievements of *mankind* are unparalleled in history.	1. The recent scientific achievements of *men and women* are unparalleled in history. 2. The recent scientific achievements of *humans* are unparalleled in history.	
The *child* is not alone in *his* language acquisition process. *He* gets significant help from *his* caregivers.	1. The *children* are not alone in their language acquisition process. *They* get significant help from *their* caregivers. 2. The *child* is not alone in *his or her* language acquisition process. *He or she* gets significant help from caregivers.	The excessive use of *he or she* makes the writing cumbersome to read. Prefer the plural pronouns as in the first example.
The child may be referred to a *pediatrician* with the expectation that he will follow up on the recommendations.	The child may be referred to a *pediatrician* with the expectation that *she or he* will follow up on the recommendations.	Alternate the order in which you write *he or she (she or he) woman or man (man or woman)*

B.2.1. Write Without Gender Biases

Incorrect	Write Correctly
The stuttering client is typically frustrated with his attempts at communication.	
Mankind has known about aphasia for a long time, though the treatment methods were unknown.	
Refer the client to a biotechnician. He will make a prosthetic device for the client.	
Hearing loss in old age affects a man's social behavior.	
Today's college student is a busy person. He hardly has time to relax.	
Giving accurate information to a client is a clinician's ethical responsibility. He never should evade it.	
The child should be treated as a total person. He should not be thought of merely as a client.	
You should refer all voice clients to a laryngologist. He should medically evaluate the clients.	

B.2.2. Write Without Prejudicial Reference to Disabilities

Describe disabilities objectively.

Avoid sentimental, evaluative, or euphemistic terms.

Put people first, not their disability.

Do not use disabilities to suggest metaphoric meanings.

Incorrect	Correct	Note
The man was a *victim* of laryngectomy.	The man had laryngectomy.	Avoid such terms as *victim, suffers from, and crippled* because they suggest negative evaluations.
The child *suffers* from severe articulation problems.	The child has a severe articulation disorder.	
The man with aphasia is *crippled.*	The man with aphasia has hemiplegia.	
The *stutterer* could not order in restaurants.	1. Mr. Jones, who stutters, could not order in restaurants. 2. A person who stutters has difficulty ordering in restaurants.	The correct versions put the persons first, not their disabilities.
The child *stutterer* did not ask questions in the classroom.	1. The child, because of her stuttering, did not ask questions in the classroom. 2. The child, who stutters, did not ask questions in the classroom.	
The *aphasic* did not recall the names.	1. The woman with aphasia did not recall the names. 2. The aphasic person did not recall the names.	The term *aphasic* is not a noun; it is an adjective.
The *wheelchaired* need access to our classrooms and clinics.	Persons in wheelchairs need access to our classrooms and clinics.	
Supervisors are *blind* to our day-to-day problems.	1. Supervisors do not see our day-to-day problems. 2. Supervisors do not appreciate our day-to-day problems.	Metaphoric use of a disability.

B.2.2. Write Without Prejudicial Reference to Disabilities

Incorrect	Write Correctly
The child was a victim of bilateral clefts of the hard palate.	
The woman suffers from dementia.	
The disabled person is crippled.	
Blind and deaf children need special methods to learn communication.	
The teachers' plea for more computers fell on deaf ears.	
This aphasic has lost her speech.	
The deaf child learned to use the sign language.	
The stutterer agreed to come for treatment.	
The dysarthric had prosodic problems.	
The paraplegic need appropriate access to buildings.	
Disabled people have rights, too.	

B.3. FORMAT OF SCIENTIFIC WRITING

B.3.1. Give Correct Margins

Margins should be 1 inch (2.54 cm) on the top, bottom, right, and left of every page. Make sure you use the specified margins on all papers you submit.

	Top 1"	
Left 1"		Right 1"
	Bottom 1"	

B.3.2. Use Appropriate Line Spacing

Double Space	Triple Space	Single Space
title page entire paper all headings all text quotations tables figure legends reference lists	before starting a major heading (optional)	no portion of a research or term paper Exception: The final versions of clinical reports and all forms of correspondence. These are always single-spaced.

B.3.3. Use Acceptable Computer Printers and Typefaces

Acceptable	Unacceptable	Note
Letter-quality printers Laser printers Ink jet printers	Dot matrix printers Exotic and ornamental typefaces Cursive typefaces Condensed type	Use typefaces that are clear and easy to read.

B.3.4. Do Not Overuse Boldface

Use bold to	Do not use bold to	Note
highlight technical or other important terms. highlight headings and subheadings.	highlight quotations	Do not use bold when italics are needed (e.g., book and journal titles).

B.3.5. Use the Recommended Type Size

The same size letters may look larger or smaller, depending on the typeface. For instance, 12 point Times Roman may be smaller than 12 point Geneva. Use your judgment.

Recommended Size	Unacceptable	Note
12 point	Very large or very small sizes	See how the printed page looks and make a judgment.

B.3.6. Use Acceptable Paper

Acceptable	Unacceptable	Note
For drafts: Ordinary computer or copy paper For the final submission: Letter size (8½ × 11"), white, nonerasable, unlined bond paper with 25% cotton content (letterhead quality)	For the final submission: typical computer paper or copy paper. (These are not 25% cotton bond.)	If cost is a factor, talk to your instructor to get a waiver.

B.3.7. Type Correctly the Title Page of a Paper for Publication

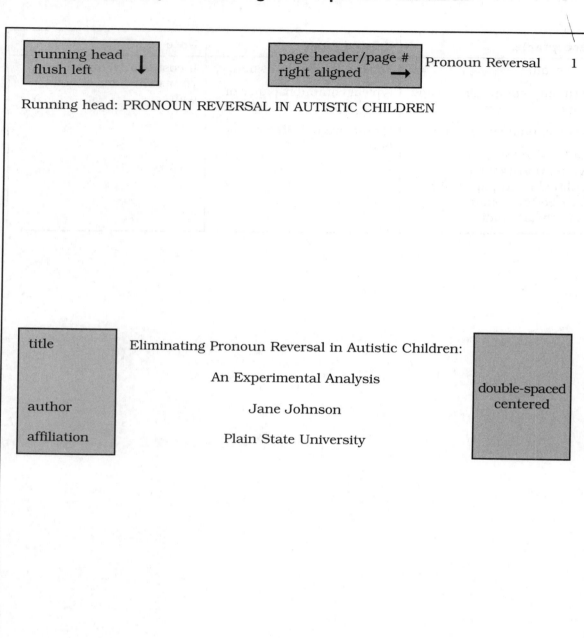

running head
flush left ↓

page header/page #
right aligned ➞   Pronoun Reversal   1

Running head: PRONOUN REVERSAL IN AUTISTIC CHILDREN

title

author

affiliation

Eliminating Pronoun Reversal in Autistic Children:

An Experimental Analysis

Jane Johnson

Plain State University

double-spaced
centered

B.3.8. Type Correctly the Title Page of a Class (Term) Paper

running head
flush left ↓

page header/page #
right aligned →

Hearing Aid Technology   1

Running head: ADVANCES IN HEARING AID TECHNOLOGY

title

author

affiliation

course

instructor

semester

Recent Advances in Hearing Aid Technology:

The Digital Processing of the Signal

Toya Tinsley

Mountain State University

CD 550 Aural Rehabilitation

Professor Melinda Malaaissonn

Spring, 1998

double-spaced
centered

B.3.9. Type the Page Header and the Running Head Correctly

Type a **page header**—a shorter version of the title—at the top right hand corner of **each page** (including the title page), except pages that contain figures. The page header is only to identify the manuscript. It is not printed in a published article.

Type a **running head** at the top of **only the first page**. A running head, although shorter than the full title, is more complete than the page header and may be printed on the right- or the left-hand pages of published articles or books.

Pronoun Reversal   1

Running head: PRONOUN REVERSAL IN AUTISTIC CHILDREN

Eliminating Pronoun Reversal in Autistic Children:

An Experimental Analysis

Jane Johnson

Plain State University

B.3.10. Write an Abstract on the Second Page

Type an abstract on the second page.
Type the word Abstract at the top, center portion of the page.
Do not indent the first line.
Type the page header and the page number on the top right-hand corner.
Double-space the abstract.
Do not exceed 960 characters (including punctuation and spaces).
Type all numbers as digits (except those that begin a sentence).

Pronoun Reversal   2

Abstract

Pronoun reversal, a persistent language problem of children with autism, has been difficult to eliminate. It has been suggested that echolalia, which is frequently observed in children with autism, may contribute to pronoun reversal. I tested this possibility by reducing echolalia with a time-out contingency and by measuring the frequency of pronoun reversal. Four children between 5 and 7 years of age, diagnosed with autism, were the subjects. I used the multiple baseline design across the four subjects. As the experimental contingency of time-out decreased the frequency of echolalia, the frequency of pronoun reversal also decreased.

B.3.11. Begin the Text on Page Three

Eliminating Pronoun Reversal in Autistic Children:

An Experimental Analysis

Among the many language characteristics of children with autism, echolalia and pronoun reversal occur frequently. **Echolalia** is the seemingly meaningless repetition of what is heard. **Pronoun reversal** refers to the frequent substitution of an appropriate personal pronoun with an inappropriate pronoun. For example, a child with autism may substitute *you* for *me* and vice versa (Johnson, 1997).

(text continued)

Note: Defined terms may be underlined, italicized, or printed in bold type. Remember, in a published article, underlined words will be converted to italics.

B.3.12. Number the Pages Correctly

Do	Do not	Note
place the page number on the top right-hand corner, one line below or five spaces to the right of the page header.	number the pages that contain figures and figure captions.	On most word processing programs, use the *Header* command to automatically insert page numbers and headers. Format page numbers as a right-aligned paragraph to print them at the end of the right margin.
number all pages of the paper consecutively, including the title page, tables, and other end materials.		
insert unnumbered pages at the end of the paper following all numbered material.		
renumber or repaginate the entire paper when you delete or add pages.	Do not give a new identity to the inserted pages (e.g., 32A, 59B).	

B.3.13. Reprint the Corrected Pages

Do	Do not	Note
reprint or retype the corrected pages.	use handwritten corrections on your paper.	Final submission should be free from distracting corrections.
	use correction paper or liquid.	

B.3.14. Use Correct Indentation

Indent	Do not indent	Note
five to seven spaces: the first line of each paragraph of the text level four headings the first line of each reference on the reference list	abstracts level three headings titles of tables legends of figures the second and subsequent lines of each reference on the reference list	Most headings and titles are **centered**. Unindented lines are typed *flush left*. **Variation:** For term papers and clinic reports, indent paragraphs by three spaces.

B.3.15. Give Correct Space or No Space After Punctuation

Correct	Number of Spaces
	One space after
Speech, language, and hearing	commas
The clinician said: "Stop!"	colons
These rules may be vague; nonetheless, you are expected to follow them!	semicolons
The data were impressive. But no one cared. He said "Let us go!" She asked, "Go where?"	punctuation marks at the end of a sentence
Penn, P. Z. (1993). Q. X. Zenkin	each period that separates initials in names
	One space between
Penn, P. Z. (1993). *Nation of Children.* New York: Infancy Press	each element in a reference list
	One space on either side of
10 – 5 is 5. (a hyphen serves as a minus sign)	a minus sign
	One space before, but no space after
The negative value was –70.	negative values
	No space after
p.m.; i.e.; U.S.	internal periods in abbreviations
The ratio is 4:1.	around colons in ratios
The book is yet-to-be published. (hyphen) The client—a professional singer—came to the clinic with hoarse voice. (dashes) (According to the APA *Manual*, typed as two hyphens --)	before or after hyphens and dashes

B.3.16. Use the Headings Within the Text Consistently

Headings are important for both the author and the reader. Thoughtfully designed headings help readers understand the material better. Scientific articles tend to have many standard headings (e.g., Method, Results, Discussion). In term papers written to fulfill class requirements, students have more freedom to use different levels and styles of headings.

Headings should be brief and direct. They should help concentrate on the topic or discussion that follows.

The number and styles of headings vary. Scientific papers have fewer headings than lengthy chapters in books. Headings in book chapters also use more appealing and creative styles than journal articles.

APA style includes up to five levels of headings. In the pages that follow, these headings are illustrated. You should select a heading style and use it consistently.

An introduction is **untitled**. A common mistake is to type *Introduction* at the beginning of a paper.

For a research proposal you submit to complete a class requirement, two levels of headings may be adequate. Use additional levels if necessary.

Journals that purport to use the APA style are not entirely faithful to all aspects of that style, especially to the levels of headings. Therefore, if you are required to follow the APA style, you must be faithful to it.

With the capabilities of your computer software and printer, you can make your headings more attractive than those in the APA style. However, do this only after your instructor approves it.

A few common variations of the APA style also are illustrated in the pages that follow. First learn the APA style and then try to be more creative.

Two Levels of Headings

Method ❶

(Centered Uppercase and Lowercase Heading)

<u>Subjects</u> ❷

(Flush Left, Underlined, Uppercase and Lowercase Side Heading)

APA style requires that you underline the level 2 heading. It will be printed as italicized. For a term paper, you may italicize it. Ask your instructor. Also, the headings in the APA style are not typed in boldface; but you may use boldface for a class paper.

An Example of Two Levels of Headings

Hearing Impairment
8

Method ❶

❷
<u>Subjects</u>

    I will select 20 children from a special class for children with hearing impairment. The children will come from middle-class families. The parents will have normal hearing.

❷
<u>Procedure</u>

    The aural rehabilitation program to be evaluated will include an initial hearing evaluation, selection and fitting of a hearing aid, and parent counseling.

Results ❶

The results of the study are presented in Table 1. As the table shows, . . .

Discussion ❶

Although many aural rehabilitation programs exist, few have been experimentally evaluated for their effectiveness. The present study shows that . . .

A Common Variation of Two Levels of Headings

METHOD ❶

❷
Subjects

❷
Materials

❷
Procedures

RESULTS ❶

DISCUSSION ❶

Note that in this variation from the APA style, the first level heading is typed in **all capitals and the second level is italicized.** (In no case do you both underline and italicize, however.) All headings are in **boldface**. Many journals use this format. The journals ASHA publishes show other variations in the way the articles are set up. Compare some of these variations with the APA style.

Three Levels of Headings

Method ❶

(Centered Uppercase and Lowercase Heading)

❷

<u>Procedure</u>

(Flush Left, Underlined, Uppercase and Lowercase Side Heading)

❸

   <u>Baselines</u>. We established the baselines with 20 stimulus items. We used a series of modeled trials and a series of evoked trials . . .

(Indented, underlined, lowercase paragraph heading ending with a period. After one space, the text is started on the same line, as typed above.)

Note: This is an APA style. Again, with your instructor's permission, you may use boldface for all headings and italicize level two and level three headings.

Four Levels of Headings

Experiment 2 ❶

(Centered Uppercase and Lowercase Heading)

Method ❷

(Centered, Underlined, Uppercase and Lowercase Heading)

❸

<u>Materials</u>

(Flush Left, Underlined, Uppercase and Lowercase Side Heading)

❹

<u>Training pictures</u>. I will prepare the training pictures that represent . . .

(Indented as for a paragraph, underlined, lowercase paragraph heading ending with a period. After one space, the text is started on the same line, as typed above.)

Note: This is an APA style. In a variation of this style that may be used in a class paper, you may use all capitals for level 1 headings, italics for the second, third, and fourth level headings, and boldface for all headings.

Five Levels of Headings

EXPERIMENT 1: MORPHOLOGIC TRAINING ❺
(CENTERED UPPERCASE HEADING)

Establishing the Target Responses ❶
(Centered Uppercase and Lowercase Heading)

<u>Method</u> ❷
(Centered, Underlined, Uppercase and Lowercase Heading)

❸
<u>Subjects</u>
(Flush Left, Underlined, Uppercase and Lowercase Side Heading)

❹
   <u>The training procedure</u>. I used the incidental training procedure. In each session . . .

   (Indented, underlined, lowercase, paragraph heading ending with a period. After two spaces, the text is started on the same line, as typed above.)

Note: This is another APA style. Vary as approved by your instructor.

Note to Student Writers

The APA heading styles are required for research papers to be submitted to a journal that uses that style. For term papers and clinical reports, you can vary the heading styles to make use of the various default styles available in computer word processors. You can create your own styles, too. Make sure, however, that deviations from the APA style are acceptable to your instructor or clinical supervisor.

Also, as noted in *B.1. Introduction to Scientific Writing*, books, including this one, do not fully conform to all aspects of the APA style. Books are uniquely designed to conform to the style of the publishing house and for esthetic purposes. Therefore, APA style exemplars are not to be determined by looking at the stylistic aspects of this or any other book.

B.3.17. Write Out Abbreviations the First Time You Use the Term and Enclose the Abbreviations in Parentheses

First Correct Citation	Subsequent Correct Citation	Note
The hearing threshold level (HTL) was measured . . .	The HTL was . . .	These audiological abbreviations need not be spelled out even the first time if an audiogram that spells them out accompanies the report or the reader is likely to know them.
A value of 100 Hertz (Hz) means that . . .	A tone of 200 Hz was presented.	
A decibel (dB) is one tenth of a Bel.	In 5 dB increments . . .	
The temporomandibular joint (TMJ) is an important joint . . .	The TMJ is important for . . .	
We measured the mean length of utterance (MLU) in syllables.	The obtained MLU values are shown in Table 1.	
The tone—a conditioned stimulus (CS)—may be presented . . .	The intensity of CS was increased.	
You must obtain your Certificate of Clinical Competence (CCC).	The American Speech-Language-Hearing Association issues the CCC in . . .	
Our professional organization is the American Speech-Language-Hearing Association (ASHA).	The president of ASHA spoke at the convention.	

B.3.18. Do Not Start a Sentence With a Lowercase Abbreviation

Incorrect	Correct	Note
dB is one tenth of a Bel.	The dB is one tenth of a Bel.	
ppb is useful in measuring the amount of pesticides in water.	The amount of the residual pesticide in water is measured in ppb.	These are the subsequent citations of the abbreviated words.

ppb = parts per billion

B.3.17. Write Out Abbreviations the First Time You Use the Team and Enclose the Abbreviations in Parentheses

Incorrect	Rewrite Correctly
The ASHA code of ethics is an important document. The members of ASHA should adhere to the code.	
In hearing evaluation, the SDT should be obtained. The (SDT) is the hearing level at which a person is just aware of speech.	
A loud noise is a UCS for startle response. The presentation of a UCS results in UCR.	
The LAD is the mechanism by which children derive the grammar of their language. Without the LAD, the child would be lost in confusion.	
In DRO, you specify the behavior that will not be reinforced. The effectiveness of DRO is well established.	
The child has a P.E. tube. Surgically implanted P.E. tubes allow for middle ear ventilation.	

ASHA: American Speech-Language-Hearing Association
SDT: Speech-detection threshold
UCS: Unconditioned stimulus; UCR: Unconditioned response
LAD: Language acquisition device
DRO: Differential reinforcement of other behavior
P.E. tube: Pressure-equalizing tube

B.3.18. Do Not Start a Sentence With a Lowercase Abbreviation

Incorrect	Write Correctly
cc, being a metric measure . . .	
lb is a popular measure in the U.S.	

cc: cubic centimeter
lb: pound

B.3.19. Do Not Write Out Units of Measurement When a Number Is Specified

Incorrect	Correct	Note
20 seconds 2 hours 20 kilograms 5 centimeters 29 percent	20 sec 2 hr 20 kg 5 cm 29%	In scientific papers, units of time and other measures are abbreviated. The units are always singular (e.g., kg, *not* kgs). Unless they are at the end of a sentence, there is no period at the end of these abbreviations. **Exception:** *in.* (for inch; a period is always added).

Note: In the noun phrase, no hyphen is used between the number and the abbreviation (20 sec); a hyphen is used in an adjectival phrase (as in *a 20-sec interval will be used*).

B.3.20. Write Out Units of Measurement When a Number Is Not Specified

Incorrect	Correct	Note
The weight was specified in kg. The specified weight was 10 kilograms.	The weight was specified in kilograms. The specified weight was 10 kg.	A specified number is always followed by an abbreviated unit of measure.
measured in cm . . . It was 10 centimeters long.	measured in centimeters . . . It was 10 cm long.	
several lb of sugar You have 10 pounds of sugar	several pounds of sugar . . . You have 10 lb of sugar.	An unspecified unit of measure is always followed by a word, not an abbreviation.
calculated the % of dysfluencies . . . The client had a 10 percent dysfluency rate.	calculated the percentage of dysfluencies . . . The client had a 10% dysfluency rate.	

B.3.21. Add the Lowercase Plural Morpheme *s* to Plural Abbreviations Without an Apostrophe

Incorrect	Correct	Note
ABR's; ECG's; EEG's; IQ's; Ed's.; vol's.	ABRs; ECGs; EEGs; IQs; Eds. (for Editors); vols.	A common mistake is to add an apostrophe

B.3.19. Do Not Write Out Units of Measurement When a Number Is Specified

Incorrect	Write Correctly
10 minute	
10 feet	
5 pounds	
5 seconds	
15 centimeters	

B.3.20. Write Out Units of Measurement When a Number Is Not Specified

Incorrect	Write Correctly
You can take several mg without side effects.	
The voice onset time of persons who stutter was slower by several ms.	

mg: milligrams
ms: milliseconds

B.3.21. Add the Lowercase Plural Morpheme s to Plural Abbreviations Without an Apostrophe

Incorrect	Write Correctly
HTL's	
MLU's	
SRT's	
FR's (for Fixed Ratio of reinforcement)	

B.3.22. With Abbreviations, Use the Period Correctly

Add periods to	Do not add periods to
Initials of names (Z. Q. Xompompin)	Capital letter abbreviations and acronyms: ASHA; APA; UNESCO; IQ.
Doctoral degree abbreviations: Ph.D., M.D., D.D.S., J.D. (*Note:* Practice varies with these degrees; some omit the period)	
Geographic names (U.S. Military)	
U.S. as an adjective (U.S. Department of Health and Human Services)	Abbreviations of state names: CA, NY
Latin abbreviations: *i.e.; vs.; a.m.; e.g.*	
Reference abbreviations: *vol.; 2nd ed.; p.* 10.	

B.3.23. Use Roman Numerals Only When It Is an Established Practice

Incorrect	Correct
Cranial nerve 4	Cranial nerve IV
Type 2 error	Type II error

B.3.24. Use Arabic Numerals for All Numbers 10 and Above

However, see exceptions under B.3.25.

Incorrect	Correct	Note
I selected eleven subjects.	I selected 11 subjects.	Numbers 10 and above are not written in words unless they start a sentence.
The client is seventy-five years old.	The client is 75 years old.	
The client met the training criterion on the fifteenth trial.	The client met the training criterion on the 15th trial.	
The client was twenty percent dysfluent.	The client was 20% dysfluent.	

B.3.22. With Abbreviations, Use the Period Correctly

Incorrect	Write Correctly
US Park Service	
Secretary, US Department of Labor	
viz	
etc	

B.3.23. Use Roman Numerals Only When It Is an Established Practice

Incorrect	Write Correctly
Cranial nerve 8	
Type one error	

B.3.24. Use Arabic Numerals for All Numbers 10 and Above

Incorrect	Write Correctly
A caseload of fifty-five is large.	
The client met the training criterion in only twelve trials.	
The client's baserate production was fifteen percent.	
There are ten clients on the waiting list.	

B.3.25. Use Numerals for All Numbers Below 10 in Specified Contexts

Generally, numerals below 10 are written out in words. There are exceptions, however. Numbers below 10 are written in numerals when they:

- are grouped for comparison with number 10 or above
- precede a unit of measurement
- represent statistical or mathematical functions
- represent time; dates; ages; sample; number of subjects in a study; scores on a scale; exact amounts of money; and items in a quantitative series

Incorrect	Correct	Note
I answered only nine out of 12 questions.	I answered only 9 out of 12 questions.	In each of these examples, a number below 10 is compared with a number 10 or above. Therefore, even the numbers below 10 are written in numerals.
Stimuli include five pictures, three toys, and 12 objects.	Stimuli include 5 pictures, 3 toys, and 12 objects.	
The ninth graders did better than the 12th graders.	The 9th graders did better than the 12th graders.	
The fourth and 15th subjects did not do well.	The 4th and the 15th subjects did not do well.	
Of the 15 clients, four dropped out of therapy.	Of the 15 clients, 4 dropped out of therapy.	
Only seven of the 20 probe responses were correct.	Only 7 of the 20 probe responses were correct.	
I used three lb of sugar.	I used 3 lb of sugar.	Numbers precede units of measurement
I took a five-mg tablet.	I took a 5-mg tablet.	
I divided it by seven.	I divided it by 7.	Numbers with statistical or mathematical functions.
A dysfluency rate of five % is high.	A dysfluency rate of 5% is high.	
The third quartile.	The 3rd quartile.	
The experiment took two weeks.	The experiment took 2 weeks.	Numbers that represent time, date, age, and so forth
I completed the degree in four years.	I completed the degree in 4 years.	
The subjects were four-year-olds.	The subjects were 4-year-olds.	
She scored six on a 7-point scale.	She scored 6 on a 7-point scale.	
Please see Table Five for details.	Please see Table 5 for details.	Number in a series (of tables and pages, in this case).
You can find this on page seven.	You can find this on page 7.	

B.3.25. Use Numerals for All Numbers Below 10 in Specified Contexts

Incorrect	Write Correctly
I scored only six out of 12 answers.	
The seventh graders did better than the 11th graders.	
The third and 12th subjects did not do well.	
Of the 17 clients, 6 needed booster treatment.	
The client's responses were correct on the seventh and 11th trials.	
I bought five kg of pesticide.	
The normal dosage is three-mg.	
Multiply this number by four.	
An error rate of seven % is unacceptable.	
I completed the study in four weeks.	
I had seven-year-olds as subjects.	
He scored five on a 7-point scale.	
Please see page nine.	
These data are presented in Figure four.	

B.3.26. Write Out in Words Numbers Below 10 Under Specified Contexts

Use this general rule, but take note of exceptions to this rule in B.3.25.
Use words instead of numerals to write numbers that are:

- not precisely measured values
- not set in comparison with numbers 10 and above
- the numbers zero and one in most (but not all) cases
- common fractions
- traditionally expressed only in words

Incorrect	Correct	Note
Such instances are few; perhaps 3 or 4.	Such instances are few; perhaps three or four.	Precise measurement is not implied.
The client repeated it 3 times.	The client repeated it three times.	
These are 4 concepts that mean the same.	These are four concepts that mean the same.	
She is the only 1 who is well prepared.	She is the only one who is well prepared.	
The client has missed 2 or 3 sessions this semester.	The client has missed two or three sessions this semester.	
After 5 imitated responses, I will fade modeling.	After five imitated responses, I will fade modeling.	*Five or eight* is not in comparison with number 10 or above
I will use 8 items for training.	I will use eight items for training.	
He got a 0 on the test.	He got a zero on the test.	the numbers *zero* and *one* in most (but not all) cases
Still, 1 response was wrong.	Still, one response was wrong. **(but,** Only 1 out of 15 was wrong).	
Do not write a 1-line sentence.	Do not write a one-line sentence.	
One 5th of the class was absent today. 1/5th of the class was absent today.	One fifth of the class was absent today.	common fractions *Note:* The second wrong example also starts the sentence with a number, another violation.
You need a 2/3 majority.	We need a two-thirds majority	
The 4th of July was a hot day.	The fourth of July was a hot day.	traditionally expressed only in words
The 10 commandments are well known.	The ten commandments are well known.	

B.3.26. Write Out in Words Numbers Below 10 Under Specified Contexts

Incorrect	Write Correctly
At any one time, 4 to 5 students can observe the sessions.	
Approximately 7 weeks of training may be needed to meet the training criterion.	
The instructor repeated it 4 times.	
These 5 terms have similar meanings.	
He is the only 1 who can be trusted.	
I will use 6 stimuli on my probe list.	
It is no fun having 0-degree temperature.	
Today, 1/4th of the class is absent.	
The *12th Night* is a play by Shakespeare.	
The original 12 Apostles were the disciples of Jesus.	

B.3.27. Write Out in Words Any Number That Begins a Sentence

Do not begin a sentence with a numeral. This rule applies to titles and headings as well.

Incorrect	Correct	Note
5 children were tested.	Five children were tested.	No sentence is started with a number written in numerals.
7 clients attended all sessions and 4 did not attend any.	Seven clients attended all sessions and 4 did not attend any.	
75 clinicians attended the workshop.	Seventy-five clinicians attended the workshop.	
15% of the school children have some form of communicative disorders.	Fifteen percent of the school children have some form of communicative disorders.	
99 Ways to Get A Grades	Ninety-nine Ways to Get A Grades	An article title

B.3.28. Combine Words and Numerals in Specified Contexts

Several constructions require a combination of words and numerals. Expressions that include large numbers (million and more) and back-to-back modifiers use a combination of words and numerals.

Incorrect	Correct	Note
The population is at least five million.	The population is at least 5 million.	A large number
We have two two-way mirrors. We have 2 2-way mirrors.	We have 2 two-way mirrors.	Back-to-back numerical modifiers.
We selected 6 9-year-olds for the study.	We selected six 9-year-olds for the study.	
I had the speech rated on 2 5-point scales.	I had the speech rated on two 5-point scales.	
Check the 1st 12 entries in the index.	Check the first 12 entries in the index.	

B.3.27. Write Out in Words Any Number That Begins a Sentence

Incorrect	Write Correctly
9 phonemes will be trained.	
39th percentile is not too impressive.	
37 children will be screened.	
80% probe response rate did not meet the criterion.	
29 Methods of Stuttering Treatment	

B.3.28. Combine Words and Numerals in Specified Contexts

Incorrect	Write Correctly
You cannot really see seven million people at one time!	
The city has only two two-way streets.	
Our research included 7 2-year-olds.	
Use 3 7-point scales for reliability.	
Check the 1st 4 items on the menu.	

B.3.29. Distinguish Between a Reference List and a Bibliography

A reference list includes the books, articles, and other sources cited in a piece of writing. The list is always attached to a paper, a book, or other form of writing. A reference list contains all that is cited and only what is cited in the text; an author who studied other sources but did not cite them, should not include them in the reference list. All research papers, term papers, theses, and other kinds of academic writing have reference citations in the text and a reference list at the end.

A bibliography is a list of all or most of the articles published on a topic. A bibliography stands alone; it may not be attached to any text.

REFERENCE CITATION WITHIN THE TEXT

B.3.30. Cite the Author's Last Name and Year of Publication in the Text

Incorrect	Correct	Note
In her study of heavyweight champions, Byson found that . . .	In her study of heavyweight champions, Byson (1993) found that . . .	The author's name is part of the narration. Therefore, only the year is in parentheses.
Ticklishson stated that humor is good medicine (1992).	Ticklishson (1992) stated that humor is good medicine.	Type the year immediately after the name.
Byson (1993) found that the reaction time of his opponents was sluggish . . . . Byson (1993) also found that . . .	Byson (1993) found that the reaction time of his opponents was sluggish . . . . Byson also found that . . .	Omit the year when the same study is referred to again within the same paragraph if it cannot be confused with another.
A study showed that boxing causes brain damage; Hali, 1992.	A study showed that boxing causes brain damage (Hali, 1992).	When the name and the year are not a part of the narrative, enclose both within parentheses.
In (1978), MacVinro was the first to show that playing tennis sharpens the tongue.	In 1978, MacVinro was the first to show that playing tennis sharpens the tongue.	If the year also is a part of the narration, do not enclose it in parentheses.

B.3.31. Cite Both Names in the Text When a Work Has Two Authors

Incorrect	Correct	Note
Tang et al., (1993) found that college courses are incomprehensible.	Tang and Lagassi (1993) found that college courses are incomprehensible.	Always cite both authors of a single work.

B.2.29. Distinguish Between a Reference List and a Bibliography

List the characteristics of a reference list and a bibliography.

A reference list is:	A bibliography is:

REFERENCE CITATION WITHIN THE TEXT

B.3.30. Cite the Author's Last Name and Year of Publication in the Text

Incorrect	Write Correctly
June John Jinkinson (1993) stated that . . .	
In (1992), Torkinson reported that . . .	
Jasperson's study has shown that . . . (1992).	
Research shows that bilingualism is enriching; Fung, 1992.	

B.3.31. Cite Both Names in the Text When a Work Has Two Authors

Reference Information	Write a Sentence Using the Information
1. Authors: Cheng and Tang Year: 1993 Study on: Elimination of phonological processes Results: Only some processes were eliminated. 2. Authors: Haniff and Chwe Year: 1992 Study on: incidence of stuttering in general population Result: about 1%.	1. End the sentence with the reference: 2. Begin the sentence with the names:

B.3.32. Cite Works With Three to Five Authors Using All the Authors' Names Only the First Time

Subsequently, cite only the first author's last name and add "et al." to it. Include the year of publication.

Incorrect	Correct	Note
In a study on head injury, Hali et al. (1993) found that . . . *(first citation)*	In a study on head injury, Hali, Byson, and Tedson (1972) found that . . . *(first citation)* The results of Hali et al. (1972) were that . . . *(subsequent citation)*	Three authors, all cited the first time. *et al.* with no period after et (not *et. al.*); neither underlined nor italicized
In their study on vocal nodules, Lordon et al., (1992) discovered that . . . *(first citation)* Lordon et al. (1992) showed that . . . *(subsequent citation)*	In their study on vocal nodules, Lordon, Fontana, Tanseko, Pendl, and Tavratino (1992) discovered that . . . *(first citation)* Lordon et al. (1992) showed that . . . *(subsequent citation)*	Five authors, all cited the first time.

B.3.33. Cite Works of Six or More Authors by Only the First Author

Follow this rule even for the first citation.

Type "et al." after the first author's last name followed by the year of publication; do not type a comma after the name when only one name is mentioned (e.g., Wang et al.; *not* Wang, et al.); add a comma when more than one name precedes et al. (e.g., Wang, Smith, et al.; *not* Wang, Smith et al.)

Incorrect	Correct	Note
Wang, Bhat, Johnson, Hernadez, Allende, Singh, and Smith (1992) have studied the effects of . . . *(first citation)*	Wang et al. (1992) have studied the effects of . . . *(first and subsequent citations).*	Add additional names only when it is necessary to distinguish works of multiple authors. (See rule B.3.34.)
Wren, Ram, Traveno, Kelly, Trudeau, and Boonthenthorpe (1993) reported that . . . *(first citation)*	Wren et al. (1993) reported that . . . *(first and subsequent citations).*	

B.3.32. Cite Works With Three to Five Authors Using All the Authors' Names Only the First Time

Show the **first** and one **subsequent** citation.

Reference Information	Write a Sentence Using the Information
1. Authors: Shanker, Shantler, Samuelson, Whau, and Mistry Year: 1989 Study: New surgical methods of closing the complete palatal cleft Results: favorable	1.
2. Authors: Southerland, Pena, and Pundit Year: 1990 Study: New methods of auditory masking Results: no improvement over existing methods	2.

B.3.33. Cite Works of Six or More Authors by Only the First Author

Reference Information	Write a Sentence Using the Information
1. Authors: Soong, Moong, Moore, Raju, McLaughlin, and Johnson Year: 1993 Study on: noise suppression by digital hearing aids Results: very effective	1.
2. Authors: Mann, Nath, Fahey, Lahey, Bohey, Johey, and Pinkerton Year: 1992 Study on: central auditory processing in persons who stutter Results: no abnormalities	2.

B.3.34. Distinguish Works of Multiple Authors Published in the Same Year

If two studies published in the same year with a different combination of three or more authors have the same first author, then cite all names if necessary; or, cite as many names as you need to distinguish the two studies.

Incorrect	Correct	Note
Lordon et al. (1997) have concluded that . . . *(subsequent citation)* *(This study had four authors: Lordon, Fontana, Tanseko, and Pendl)* Lordon et al. (1997) also have concluded that . . . *(subsequent citation)* *(A different study published in the same year that had a different combination of four authors: Lordon, Fontana, Tanseko, and Jensen)*	Lordon, Fontana, Tanseko, and Pendl (1997) showed that . . . Lordon, Fontana, Tanseko, and Pendl (1997) have concluded that . . . *(all names of this study cited each time)* Lordon, Fontana, Tanseko, and Jensen (1997) also reported that . . . Lordon, Fontana, Tanseko, and Jensen (1997) also have concluded that . . . *(all names of this other study also cited each time)*	Even in subsequent citations, all authors are cited to distinguish the two studies. If not, the two studies would be confused as they both abbreviate to Lordon et al. (1997).
Tinsonn et al. (1996) have found no significant difference. *(This study had seven authors: Tinsonn, Fung, Haniff, Chwe, Boonthenthorpe, Alvarado, and Smith)* Tinsonn et al. (1996) did not find the method effective. *(This study had six authors: Tinsonn, Fung, Mendoza, Kumar, Azevedo, and Alfonso)*	Tinsonn, Fung, et al. (1996) have found no significant difference. Tinsonn, Fung, Mendoza, et al. (1996) did not find the method effective.	The two studies had six or more authors, published in the same year. The addition of a third name distinguishes the two studies. A comma is added to the last name (before et al.) because of multiple names.

B.3.34. Distinguish Works of Multiple Authors Published in the Same Year

Use the names of as many authors as needed to distinguish the two studies.

Reference Information	Write a Sentence Using the Information
1. Authors: Rodriguez, Ford, Williams, Johnson, and Benson Year: 1998 Study: effects of modeling on autistic children's speech Result: modeling increased children's echolalia	1.
2. Authors: Rodriguez, Ford, Williams, Bennet, Bickley, Shekar, and Shinson Year: 1998 Study: assessment of language problems of children with mental retardation Results: numerous pragmatic problems	2.

B.3.35. Join Multiple Names With *and* or *&*

Join the names with *and* when the citation is part of the narrative.
Join the names with & (ampersand) when the citation is in parentheses.

Incorrect	Correct	Note
A survey study of Hecker & Donnors (1995) showed that crashing into each other is a profitable sport.	A survey study of Hecker and Donnors (1995) showed that crashing into each other is a profitable sport.	The names are a part of the narrative. Hence, the conjunction *and* is used.
It has been shown that the frequency of spitting on the field is related to the number of hits (Rosen and Tanseko, 1998).	It has been shown that the frequency of spitting on the field is related to the number of hits (Rosen & Tanseko, 1998).	The names are in parentheses. Hence, the *ampersand* is used.

B.3.36. Cite Multiple Authors With the Same Last Name With Their Initials Every Time They Are Cited

Follow this rule even if the years are different.

Incorrect	Correct	Note
Connors (1992) and Connors (1998) reported that . . .	Z. X. Connors (1992) and Q. X. Connors (1998) reported that . . .	The added initials help distinguish the studies.
As discussed by Z. X. Connors et al. (1994) and Connors (1994) . . .	As discussed by Z. X. Connors et al. (1994) and Q. X. Connors (1994) . . .	

B.3.35. Join Multiple Names With *and* or *&*

Reference Information	Write a Sentence Using the Information
1. Part of narration Authors: Gimmick and Himmick Year: 1993 Study: the relationship between screaming and vocal nodules Results: positive relationship	1.
2. Citation in parentheses Authors: Byson and Lyson Year: 1992 Study: programming maintenance Results: possible to program maintenance	2.

B.3.36. Cite Multiple Authors With the Same Last Name With Their Initials Every Time They Are Cited

Reference Information	Write a Sentence Using the Information
Authors: B. D. Quayle (1992) and Z. Q. Quayle (1993) Study: variations in spelling the same word Results: discovered a variety of ways to spell the same word	
Authors: A. B. Perot et al. (1991) and B. C. Perot (1992) Study: how to reduce budget deficits Results: no way	

B.3.37. Cite Multiple Works of the Same Author in a Temporally Ascending Order

Although you type multiple years, **do not** use the conjunction *and* before the final year (1989, 1990, 1992; but **not**, 1989, 1990, and 1992).

Incorrect	Correct	Note
Studies show that the more exciting the game, the greater the injury to vocal cords (Fontana, 1987, in press, 1992, 1990).	Studies show that the more exciting the game, the greater the injury to vocal cords (Fontana 1987, 1990, 1992, in press).	The *in press* citation is always the most recent.
Studies of Tonsiko and Travlatinova (1992, 1989, 1987, 1986) have shown that verbal abuse is a common locker room strategy.	Studies of Tonsiko and Travlatinova (1986, 1987, 1989, 1992) have shown that verbal abuse is a common locker room strategy.	The incorrect version is in the descending temporal order of publication.
Data suggest that the yells that induce vocal nodules excite the players (Rosery & Ruthery, 1981; 1978; 1975).	Data suggest that the yells that induce vocal nodules excite the players (Rosery & Ruthery, 1975, 1978, 1981).	Reference in parenthesis with the correct ascending order.

B.3.38. Attach Alphabetical Suffixes to the Same Author's Multiple Publications in the Same Year

Repeat the year, do not affix a, b, c, and so forth to year typed only once (1989a, 1989b, 1989c; but **not** 1989a, b, c).

In assigning a, b, c, and so forth to studies published in the same year, use the alphabetical order of the first word of titles of articles.

Incorrect	Correct	Note
Several studies by Johnson (1975-1, 1975-2, 1975-3, in press-1, in press-2) have shown that . . .	Several studies (Johnson, 1975a, 1975b, 1975c, in press—a, in press—b) have shown that . . .	Multiple *in press* entries also take a, b, c, and so forth.
Studies have shown that ball game watching increases brain size (Fontana, 1988-1, 1988-2, 1999-1, 1999-2, in press-1, in press-2; Tanseko, 1985-1, 1985-2, 1985-3, 1988-1, 1988-2).	Studies have shown that ball game watching increases brain size (Fontana, 1988a, 1988b, 1999a, 1999b, in press—a, in press—b; Tanseko, 1985a, 1985b, 1985c, 1988a, 1988b).	Multiple authors, each publishing multiple studies in two years; references in parentheses.

B.3.37. Cite Multiple Works of the Same Author in a Temporally Ascending Order

Reference Information	Write a Sentence Using the Information
Author: McVinro Studies on: treatment of hoarse voice Studies published in: 1982, 1992, 1991, 1989	Include the author's name in your narration.
Author: Moncure and Sincure Studies on: bilingual-bicultural issues Studies published in: 1993, 1986, 1989, 1991	Enclose the authors' names in parentheses.
Author: Foresight Studies on: Future professional issues Studies published in: 1986, 1993, 1992, 1989, 1987.	Enclose the author's name in parentheses.

B.3.38. Attach Alphabetical Suffixes to the Same Author's Multiple Publications in the Same Year

Reference Information	Write a Sentence Using the Information
Author: Sharp Studies: advances in cochlear implants Published: four in 1982.	Write the author's name as part of your narration.
Author: Bulltit Studies: dysphagia assessment techniques Published: three in 1992, two in 1993 Author: Hiltit Studies: dysphagia assessment techniques Published: two in 1989; two in 1992.	Cite the two authors and their publications in parentheses.

B.3.39. Within Parentheses, Arrange the Last Names of Multiple Authors in Alphabetical Order

Use the last name of the first author to determine the alphabetical order.
Separate each name with a semicolon.
Do not type *and* or & before the last citation.

Incorrect	Correct	Note
(Zoom, 1990; Began, 1989; Push, 1985; Lord, 1980)	(Began, 1989; Lord, 1980; Push, 1985; Zoom, 1990)	Follow the alphabetical, not temporal, order.
(Push & Twink, 1991; Began & Quinn, 1980; Lord, Horde, & Board, 1975).	(Began & Quinn, 1980; Lord, Horde, & Board, 1975; Push & Twink, 1991).	The last name of the first author of a study determines the alphabetical order. The names of multiple authors are joined by an ampersand.
(Benson, 1989; Dinson, 1992; Henson, 1990; Nelson, 1986; and, Olsen, 1980).	(Benson, 1989; Dinson, 1992; Henson, 1990; Nelson, 1986; Olsen, 1980).	No *and* before the last entry.
(Bloodstein, 1967; Epstein, 1975; Fonstein, 1990; & Konstein, 1993)	(Bloodstein, 1967; Epstein, 1975; Fonstein, 1990; Konstein, 1993)	No *ampersand* before the last entry.

B.3.39. Within Parentheses, Arrange the Last Names of Multiple Authors in Alphabetical Order

Reference Information	Cite the Names Within Parentheses
Authors: Thompson, 1992 Johnson, 1993 Able, 1975 Quinn, 1993	
Authors: Zonks and Gonks, 1993 Banks and Atkins, 1990 Atkins, 1960 Kinson, 1992	
Authors: Bayle, 1997 Timson, 1996 Xenon, 1998 Lyson, 1994	

┌───┐
│   **REFERENCE LIST**   │
└───┘

B.3.40. Begin the Reference List on a New Page With a Centered, Uppercase, and Lowercase Heading

Double space the entire Reference List.

Pronoun Reversal   21

┌──────────────┐
│ double space │
└──────────────┘

References

    Able, T. K. (1990). <u>The autistic children: New directions</u>. New York: Sapson Press.

    Babble, B. B. (1997). The negative effects of modeling on echolalia. <u>Journal of Autism, 10</u>, 19–25.

    Sunson, K. J. (1994). <u>Foundations of educational research</u>. Bend, IN: Prince Publishing.

Note that the preceding examples follow the APA 4th edition format. You will find, however, the following 3rd edition format in most printed journals, including several that purport to use the current APA format:

Able, T. K. (1990). *The autistic children: New directions.* New York: Sapson Press.

Babble, B. B. (1997). The negative effects of modeling on echolalia. *Journal of Autism, 10,* 19–25.

Note that the preceding examples use italics and single spacing because that is how they appear in print.

If your instructor approves it, you may use italics in term papers; your print-out will look more attractive and professional (double-spaced and the first line indented as in the APA 4th edition style):

    Able, T. K. (1990). *The autistic children: New directions.* New York: Sapson Press.

    Babble, B. B. (1997). The negative effects of modeling on echolalia. *Journal of Autism, 10,* 19–25.

REFERENCE LIST

B.3.40. Begin the Reference List on a New Page With a Centered, Uppercase, and Lowercase Heading

Write a page header, an arbitrarily selected page number, and the word *references* with the right characters and in the correct position.

B.3.41. In the Reference List, Arrange References in Alphabetical Order

- Use the last name to determine the alphabetical order.
- Alphabetize the names of multiple authors by the surname of the first author.
- Alphabetize names letter by letter, but exclude the initials.
- Arrange prefixes in their strict alphabetical order. Ignore an apostrophe attached to a prefix (M').
- Consult the biographical section of *Webster's New Collegiate Dictionary* to find the order in which surnames with articles and prepositions are arranged (names with *de, la, du, von*, etc.).
- When listing several works by the same author, but some with and some without co-authors, start with those works that do not have co-authors.
- Alphabetize the second and subsequent authors, too.

Incorrect	Correct	Note
McNeil Macmillan	Macmillan McNeil	*Mac* precedes *Mc*
Thomson, A. B. Thomas, Z. X.	Thomas, Z. X. Thomson, A. B.	Alphabetized letter-by-letter. Ignore the initials.
Tonseko, K. J., & Fontana, P. J. (1982) Tonseko, K. J., & Lordon, T. P. (1984) Tonseko, K. J. (1988) Tonseko, K. J. (1985)	Tonseko, K. J. (1985) Tonseko, K. J. (1988) Tonseko, K. J., & Fontana, P. J. (1982) Tonseko, K. J., & Lordon, T. P. (1984)	Enter the single author first. Alphabetize the second authors, too: *Tonseko & Fontana before Tonseko & Lordon*

B.3.42. Arrange Multiple Works of the Same Single Author From the Earliest to the Latest Year

Incorrect	Correct	Note
Able, P. J. (1993) Able, P. J. (1992) Able, P. J. (1989)	Able, P. J. (1989) Able, P. J. (1992) Able, P. J. (1993)	For each single author, arrange the works from the earliest to the latest year.
Benson, L. S. (1992) Benson, L. S. (1982) Benson, L. S. (1972)	Benson, L. S. (1972) Benson, L. S. (1982) Benson, L. S. (1992)	

B.3.41. In the Reference List, Arrange References in Alphabetical Order

Reference Information	Arrange the Names Alphabetically
McMinnan McDonald McFarrin Van Riper Axelrod Herbert Hernadez Alvarado von Kirk de Klerk	

B.3.42. Arrange Multiple Works of the Same Single Author From the Earliest to the Latest Year

Reference Information	Arrange the Names in the Correct Order
Larson, K. (1988) Larson, K. (1986) Larson, K. (1980)	
McDonald, P. (1993) McDonald, P. (1975) McDonald, P. (1974)	

B.3.43. Alphabetize the Titles of Several Works of the Same Author Published in the Same Year

In alphabetizing the titles, ignore the articles *A* and *The* at the beginning of the title.

Attach the lowercase letters a, b, c, and so forth to the year of publication.

(Arrange the multiple works of the same author, each published in a different year, in a temporally ascending order; see B.3.37.)

Incorrect	Correct	Note
Lagassi, A. R. (1991a). Problems of clay courts. Lagassi, A. R. (1991b). Advantages of short-handled rackets.	Lagassi, A. R. (1991a). Advantages of short-handled rackets. Lagassi, A. R. (1991b). Problems of clay courts.	The first words of the title determine the order: *Advantages* precedes *Problems*.
Massood, P. T. (1992a). Some advantages of the circular paper clips. Massood, P. T. (1992b). The case of the missing paper clip.	Massood, P. T. (1992a). The case of the missing paper clip. Massood, P. T. (1992b). Some advantages of the circular paper clips.	The article *The* is ignored in arranging these two entries.

B.3.44. Alphabetize the Different Authors With the Same Last Name According to Their Initials

Incorrect	Correct	Note
Able, Q. T. (1993) Able, A. A. (1982)	Able, A. A. (1982) Able, Q. T. (1993)	The year of publication does not matter
Tavratinova, S. N. (1987) Tavratinova, B. D. (1993)	Tavratinova, B. D. (1987) Tavratinova, S. N. (1993)	

B.3.43. Alphabetize the Titles of Several Works of the Same Author Published in the Same Year

Reference Information	Alphabetize According to the Titles
Belwae, T. P. (1989a). A potential explanation of muddy football fields. Belwae, T. P. (1989b). Crashing and winning: The cultural underpinnings of football.	
Cisnero, S. M. (1990a). Cities in decay. Cisnero, S. M. (1990b). Banking on the neighborhood.	

B.3.44. Alphabetize the Different Authors With the Same Last Name According to Their Initials

Reference Information	Alphabetize According to the Initials
Nelson, Z. T. (1988) Nelson, B. S. (1990) Nelson, A. P. (1986)	
Ramig, L. T. (1993) Ramig, C. C. (1990) Ramig, B. D. (1991)	

B.3.45. Indent the First Line of Each Reference Entry by Five to Seven Spaces and Type the Second and Subsequent Lines Flush Left

- Note that paragraph indentation for reference entries is not followed by several journals that purport to follow the APA style.
- The APA Manual suggests five to seven spaces for paragraph indent. If you are not required to follow this guideline, indent no more than 5 spaces; with some larger fonts, even three spaces may be adequate.

Incorrect	Correct	Note
Lagassi, A. R. (1991a). Problems of clay courts Lagassi, A. R. (1991b). Advantages of short-handled rackets.	Lagassi, A. R. (1991a). Advantages of short-handled rackets. Lagassi, A. R. (1991b). Problems of clay courts.	Indent the first line by five to seven spaces.
Massood, P. T. (1992a). Some advantages of the circular paper clips. Massood, P. T. (1992b). The case of the missing paper clip.	Massood, P. T. (1992a). The case of the missing paper clip. Massood, P. T. (1992b). Some advantages of the circular paper clips.	Type flush left the second and subsequent lines.

B.3.46. Use the Specified Abbreviations in Reference Lists

Abbreviation	For	Note
chap.	chapter	Lowercase abbreviations.
ed.	edition	
rev. ed.	revised edition	
2nd ed.	second edition	
Ed. (Eds.)	Editor (Editors)	(Eds.) period within the closing parenthesis.
Trans.	Translator(s)	The same abbreviation for the singular or plural.
p. (pp.)	page (pages)	Lowercase.
Vol.	Volume	Uppercase; as in Vol. 7 of a journal or book.
vols.	volumes	Lowercase for the plural *volumes*.
No.	Number	Uppercase; do not type # for number.
Pt.	Part	Uppercase.
Tech. Rep.	Technical Report	Both the abbreviated words in uppercase.
Suppl.	Supplement	Uppercase.

B.3.45. Indent the First Line of Each Reference Entry by Five to Seven Spaces and Type the Second and Subsequent Lines Flush Left

Incorrect	Rewrite Correctly
Sherma, P. K. (1989). The influence of the mother's vocabulary on the child's language acquisition. Tackle, K. K. (1990). Tackle football and the moral fiber.	

B.3.46. Use the Specified Abbreviations in Reference Lists

Unabbreviated	Write the Correct Abbreviation
chapter	
edition	
revised edition	
second edition	
Editor (Editors)	
Translator(s)	
page (pages)	
Volume	
volumes	
Number	
Part	
Technical Report	
Supplement	

SELECTED EXAMPLES OF REFERENCES

See The APA *Manual* (1994) for other examples.

B.3.47. Journal Articles in Reference Lists

- Give one space after the last initial. Type a period after the year in parentheses. Give one space before starting the article title.
- Type a coma after the last initial of the first author and join the names of two authors with an ampersand (&).
- Give one space before the journal name is typed.
- Capitalize all important words of the journal name; do not abbreviate journal titles; and underline the entire title. *If variation from this APA format is acceptable to your instructor, italicize what is supposed to be underlined.*
- Underline the volume number, but do not type the word *volume* or its abbreviation.
- Enter the page number or numbers as the last entry without *p.* or *pp.*
- For an article in press, do not give date, volume number, or page number. Replace the year of publication with the words "in press."
- Indent five to seven spaces from the left-hand margin for the first line of each reference.

Correct	Note
Bultit, B. S., Airhead, E. H., & Longwind, H. A. (1990). Intervening variables in human behavior: Thirty years of theorizing. <u>Journal of Theories Unlimited, 98</u>, 3–78.	A comma and a space separate each name.
Hazelnut, L. M., & Beachnut P. M. (in press). Nutty theories in naughty disciplines. <u>Journal of Speculative Psychology</u>.	A coma precedes an ampersand.
Lordon, M. S. (1987). The offensive tactics on the football field and delayed aphasic symptoms. <u>Journal of Speech and Hearing Disorders, 42</u>, 50–58.	One space separates the year and the article title. The journal title and the volume number are underlined. Underlined material will be converted to italics in a published article.
McVenro, J. P. (1990). The relation between umpire judgments and player verbal outbursts. <u>Journal of Verbal Abuse, 50</u>, 230–240.	

Note: These printed exemplars are not double-spaced; but your typed references should be.

SELECTED EXAMPLES OF REFERENCES

B.3.47. Journal Articles in Reference Lists

Reference Information	Correctly Write the References
Author: P. T. Lang Year: 1992 Article Title: The grammar of American Sign Language. Journal: Journal of Nonverbal Communication. Volume: 10 Pages: 15–25.	
Author: S. L. Nunez Year: in press Article Title: Models of counseling in speech and hearing. Journal: American Journal of Speech-Language Pathology.	
Authors: K. K. Rimm and B. B. Brimm Year: 1989 Article Title: The relation between maternal intonation and the child's singing ability Journal: Journal of Music Therapy Volume: 12 Pages: 13–23	

B.3.48. Books in Reference Lists

- Underline the title of the book. *If variation from this APA format is acceptable, italicize the title.* Capitalize only the first letter of the title and subtitle.
- Give one space between the year and the title, and between the title and the place of publication.
- Type the abbreviated word *Jr.* after the last initial, if applicable.
- Type the abbreviated edition number (2nd ed.) or the words "rev. ed." (for revised edition) after the title and place within parentheses.
- Type the name of the city of the publisher.
- If the city is not well-known or could be confused with another location, type the abbreviated name of the state. Use the U.S. Postal Service abbreviations for the states.
- Type the publishing company's name exactly as it appears in the book being referenced.
- For books written and published by corporations, agencies, or associations, type the word "Author" for the publisher.

Correct	Note
American Psychological Association. (1994). <u>Publication manual of the American Psychological Association</u> (4th ed.). Washington, DC: Author.	The publisher and the author are the same (a corporate author). DC is added to Washington because it could be confused with the state of Washington.
Boczquats, N. S. (1998). <u>Oceanography and communication: A new frontier</u>. Chicago: Blue Heaven Press.	One space separates: the year and the title and the title and the place of publication.
Histrionik, K. L., Jr., & Stoic, P. L. (1995). <u>Neurotic behavior</u> (2nd ed.). Los Angeles: Angeles Publishing Company.	The book edition in parentheses; not italicized.
Null, B. D. (1998). <u>Numbers in civilization</u> (rev. ed.). New York: Sappleton.	(rev. ed.) for revised edition.
Blinton, W., & Blinton, H. (1997). <u>Hope for America</u>. Hope, AR: Optimist Press.	The state abbreviation is added because the city is not well-known. A colon—not a period—follows the state abbreviation.

B.3.48. Books in Reference Lists

Reference Information	Correctly Write the References
Author: K. D. Wong Title: Bilingual Speech-Language Pathology Year: 1998 Edition: Second Publisher: Word Publishing Company City: Ames, Iowa	
Authors: S. S. Simms, T. T. Tinns, and K. K. Kimms Title: Education of Children with Central Auditory Problems Edition: Revised Year: 1997 Publisher: Nelson Publishers City: New York, New York	
Author: N. C. Gordimeir Title: Hearing Aids of the Future Year: 1929 Publisher: The Future Press City: Hazleton, Tennessee	
Author: American Speech-Language-Hearing Association Title: Your Professional Organization Year: 1998 City: Rockville Pike, Maryland Publisher: American Speech-Language-Hearing Association	

B.3.49. Edited Books and Chapters in Edited Books in Reference Lists

- Type in parentheses the abbreviated word (Ed.) for one editor or (Eds.) for multiple editors.
- Type (ed.) for an edition of a book.
- Place the author's initials at the end of the surname (*as usual*).
- Place the editor's initials at the beginning, not the end of the surname (*not as usual*).
- Type the pages of the chapter after the title and within parentheses.

Correct	Note
Baker, K. V. (1996). The unknown and the unconscious. In C. Hart (Ed.), <u>Unknown and inaccessible states of consciousness</u> (pp. 305–395). New York: Mystery Publishing House.	In the text, the author of the chapter, not the editor of the book, is cited (Baker, 1986, not Hart, 1986). Author's initials and the editor's initials are in reversed positions. The page numbers are for the cited author's chapter only.
Hunt, C. P., & Holms, G. S. (Eds.). (1998). <u>Mysteries of mental events</u>. Clovis, CA: Invisible Publishers.	This reference is for an entire edited book. (Eds.) for Editors
Xong, K. C. (Ed.). (1990). <u>Split brain is just as good</u>. Los Angeles: NeuroPress.	(Ed.) for Editor

B.3.50. Reports From Organizations and Government Agencies in Reference Lists

Correct	Note
National Child Health and Human Development. (1910). <u>How not to write research proposals</u> (DHHS Publication No. QRS-00910). Washington, DC: U.S. Government Printing Office.	"Publication No," "Report No," and so forth are in parentheses.
Norm, J. J. (1989). <u>Invariably fixed stages of cognitive development</u> (Report No. 15). Washington, DC: National Cognition Association.	The period is typed after the closing parenthesis; no period is typed at the end of the actual title of the report.

B.3.49. Edited Books and Chapters in Edited Books in Reference Lists

Reference Information	Correctly Write the References
Editors: L. B. Johns and R. K. Bangs Title: Professional Issues in Speech-Language Pathology Year: 1998 Publisher: College Press City: Los Angeles	
Author: N. O. Jackson Chapter title: Speech-language pathologist and the bilingual child Year: 1997 Pages: 135-175 Book title: Education in the Next Century Editors: A. K. Cantor and B. L. Bantor Publisher: Century Press City: Portland, Oregon	

B.3.50. Reports From Organizations and Government Agencies in Reference Lists

Reference Information	Correctly Write the References
Organization: National Institute of Public Health (NIPH) Year: 1993 Title of Publication: Threats to Public Health Publication #PQ-01-S25 City: Washington, DC From: U. S. Government Printing Press	
Author: S. L. Beans Title: Brain and Behavior Year: 1990 Publisher: National Neuroscience Association Report #67 City: Baltimore, Maryland	

B.3.51. Proceedings of Conferences and Conventions in Reference Lists

Correct	Note
Peacock, P. L., & Lyon, A. D. (1990). Cooperation among the animal kingdoms of the world. In E. L. Phant & H. I. Pottoms (Eds.), <u>Proceedings of the Ninety Fourth International Symposium of the Animal Kingdom</u> (pp. 23-57). Boston: Cobra Press.	The title of the paper is not underlined, but the title of the proceedings published as a book is.

B.3.52. Convention Presentations in Reference Lists

Correct	Note
Idlemann, P. S. (1983, November). <u>Variables related to doing nothing</u>. Paper presented at the Annual Meeting of the American Anti-workaholic Association, Bullhead City, AZ.	"Meeting," "convention," and so forth should be accurate. Underline the title of presentation. Give the month in parentheses. End with the name of the city and the state abbreviation.
Hernandez, K. S. (1992, November). <u>Caseload issues in public schools</u>. Paper presented at the Annual Convention of the American Speech-Language-Hearing Association, San Antonio, TX.	

B.3.53. Unpublished Articles, Theses, or Dissertations in Reference Lists

Correct	Note
Dimm, B. J. (1995). <u>Why some articles do not get published</u>. Unpublished manuscript.	Underline the title.
Brightly, B. B. (1997). <u>The complex relationship between self-image, hair color, and academic learning in children from low, medium, and high income levels</u>. Unpublished master's thesis, Sharp College of Education, Needles, CA.	The name of the university, the city, and the state abbreviation end the citation.
Smiley, S. S. (1985). <u>Variables related to early or late toilet training and the frequency of smiling in high school classrooms</u>. Unpublished doctoral dissertation, Haywire University, Lynn, OH.	

B.3.51. Proceedings of Conferences and Conventions in Reference Lists

Reference Information	Correctly Write the References
Author: D. V. Quietson Paper: Hearing impairment in rock musicians Pages: 87-97 Title of the book: Proceedings of the 10th national symposium on noise and hearing loss Editors of the book: C. D. Noysman and F. S. Loudman Year: 1990 City: Centralia, Illinois Publisher: Peace Press	

B.3.52. Convention Presentations in Reference Lists

Reference Information	Correctly Write the References
Author: B. J. Beans Paper: A new method of scoring language samples Presented at: National Convention of the American Speech-Language-Hearing Association Date: November, 1990 City: Atlanta, Georgia	

B.3.53. Unpublished Articles, Theses, or Dissertations in Reference Lists

Reference Information	Correctly Write the References
Author: T. K. Henkly Unpublished Article: How to get published in speech and hearing	
Author: G. V. Gyon M.A. thesis: Evaluation of an early language intervention package Year: 1990 University: Downstate University City: Rocks, New Jersey	

B.3.54. Cite the Electronic Sources Correctly

There is no universally accepted standard on citing electronic sources (database, World Wide Web or the Internet, e-mail, and so forth). The APA *Manual* recommends the style described by Xia Li and Nancy Crane (1993) in their book, *Electronic style: A guide to citing electronic information* (Westport, CT: Meckler). The following examples are based on this guide.

In citing electronic sources:

- do not add a period, even at the end of a sentence, if there is no period in the address, data path, or directory
- use lowercase letters, even for the initial letter of words that start a sentence, if the address, data path, or directory is written that way
- do not add typical punctuation marks that are not a part of the address, data path, or directory
- generally, if a source (e.g., a journal) has a printed version (as most do) and an on-line version, cite the source *you consulted;* it may be preferable to cite the printed source if that is more commonly available, however

Basic formats for:

- **Individual works, FTP:** Author. (date). *Title* (edition), [Type of medium]. Available: FTP: Directory: File:
- **Individual works, Telnet:** Author. (date). *Title* (edition), [Type of medium]. Available Telnet: Directory: File:
- **Journal articles in databases:** Author. (year, month). Title. Journal [Type of medium], volume, pages. Available: give information sufficient to retrieve the article.
- **Part of a work (e.g., chapters in a book):** Author. (date). Title In *Source* (edition), [Type of medium]. Available: FTP: Directory: File: (Complete information needed to retrieve the material).
- Entire publication (e.g., an entire journal on the Internet): *Journal Title* [Type of Medium]. Available: give information sufficient to retrieve the article.

Examples follow

B.3.55. Cite Correctly an Individual Work With an FTP (File Transfer Protocol)

Basic format for **Individual works, FTP:** Author. (date). *Title* (edition), [Type of medium]. Available: FTP: Directory: File:

Correct	Note
Zenson, B. P. (1996). *Zen and the art of Cyberspace* (2nd ed.), [Online]. Available FTP: quake.think.com Directory:pub/etext/1996 File: zen15txt	Single author of a book Pay attention to capitalization and punctuation
Ethernetton, A., Emaylon, B., Onlineson, Q. (1997). *BELCHY manual* [Online]. Available FTP: FTP QUICHE.CS.MCGILL.CA Directory: ARCHIE/DOC File: ARCHIE.MAN.TXT	Multiple authors Uppercase letters in the address
Why women voters abandoned me [Speech from George Bush's Presidential Papers], [Online]. (1992, September 2). Available FTP: nptn.org Directory: pub/campaign.92/bush.dir File: b99.txt	Type correctly parentheses and brackets
King, M. L. (1963, August). *I have a dream* [Online]. Available FTP: mrcnext.cso.uiuc.edu Directory: gutenberg/freenet File: i-have-a-dream	The date is part of the source

B.3.56. Cite Correctly an Individual Work on Telnet

Basic format for **Individual works, Telnet:** Author. (date). *Title* (edition), [Type of medium]. Available Telnet: Directory: File:

Correct	Note
Periodic table of elements [Online]. (1992). Available Telnet: gopher2.tc.umn.edu Directory: Libraries/Reference Works File: Periodic Table of Elements	The title is italicized whereas the same file name is not; also, note the difference in capitalization
Shakespeare, W. (No date). Hamlet (Arthur Bullen's Stratford Town Edition), [Online]. Available Telnet: Library.Dartmouth.edu Directory: Shakespeare Plays File: Hamlet	Type (No date) when the date of publication is not given in the source

B.3.57. Cite Correctly a Journal Article in a Database

Basic format for **Journal articles in databases:** Author. (year, month). Title. Journal [Type of medium], volume, pages. Available: give information sufficient to retrieve the article.

Correct	Note
Cyberson, C. K. (1997). Exceptional children on a unique cybertour. *Journal of Uniquetours* [Online], *58*, 300-325. Available: DIALOG File: Health Periodicals Database (149) Item: 11920808	The name of the journal and the volume number are italicized as for a printed source
Johnson, M., & Benson, K. (1996). So what is new on the Internet? New England Journal of the Internet [Online], *4*, 101ff. Available: LEXIS Library: INTREV File: ALLREV	When the ending page number is not known, type ff after the beginning page number (e.g., 101ff) to mean "and following pages"
National Aids Information Clearinghouse. (1997, January 29). Guidelines to prevent the spread of AIDS. Morbidity and Mortality Weekly Report [Online], 37 (Suppl. s-2), 1-14. Available: BRS/After Dark File: Combined health Information Data Base (CHID) Item: SA85006723	Corporate author
Jensen, K. (1996). Teaching courses on a Website. *CPRE* [Online], *2*,(6). Available FTP: ftp.gtf.org. Directory: pub/journals Files: core1.08	No page number; therefore, it is important to give accurate volume and issue number.
Hanson, T. R. (1996, April). How to write an article for electronic media. *Journal of Electronic Media*, [Online], 3(1). Available: gopher2.tc.umn.edu Directory: Libraries/Newspapers, Magazines, and Newsletters/Literary Journals/DragonZine/Vol. 5 File: N.01 03-20-96	A journal available on Telnet

B.3.58. Cite Correctly a Part of a Work From an Electronic Source

Basic format for **Part of a Work** (e.g., chapters in a book): Author. (date). Title In *Source* (edition), [Type of medium]. Available: FTP: Directory: File: (Complete information needed to retrieve the material)

Correct	Note
Peekson, P. P., Melson, M. M., & Toolson, T. T. (1997). What to do when you do not want to do anything. In *Handbook of Idleness* [Online]. Available: QPT/AfterNoon File: Handbook of Idleness (QWSS) Item: 101-132	Page numbers often unknown or unspecified; therefore, the file and the item numbers are important; if known, specify the page numbers after the book title within parentheses.
Compaq has a solution for educators. (1996, June 2). In *Dow Jones News.* [Online]. Available: Dow Jones News/Retrieval Service File: QUICK	No author identified

B.3.59. Cite Correctly an Entire Journal in a Database

Basic format for **Entire Journal:** *Journal Title* [Type of Medium]. Available: give information sufficient to retrieve the article.

Correct	Note
Journal of Applied Behavior Analysis [Online]. Available: http://www.envmed.rochester.edu/wwwrap/behavior/jaba/jabahome.htm *Journal of Applied Behavior Analysis and Therapy* [Online]. Available: http://sage.und.nodak.edu./org/jBAT/jbatinfo.html	Two journals on the Internet

B.3.60. Cite Correctly an Entire Thesis or Dissertation in a Database

Basic format for **Entire Thesis or dissertation:** Author. (date). Title of Thesis/ Dissertation (Master's thesis/Doctoral dissertation, University), [Type of Medium]. Available: give information sufficient to retrieve the article.

Correct	Note
Wishbone, K. V. (1996). *The innate ability to sleep in the classroom* (Master's thesis, University of Minerva, Minerva, Minnesota), [Online]. Available FTP:150.133.715 Directory: pub/education File: josephus.Zip	A master's thesis; the same format for a doctoral dissertation

Note to Students Working on Theses or Dissertations

The graduate schools of most universities have a set of guidelines on the preparation of theses and dissertations. Even the departments of communicative disorders that accept the APA style may have special guidelines that deviate in certain respects from the APA style. Therefore, students should consult both the APA style and the guidelines of their department and the graduate school.

B.4. FORMATS OF RESEARCH PAPERS

B.4.1. PARTS OF A RESEARCH PAPER

Printed Notes	Class Notes

ABSTRACT

An abstract is a brief description of the problems, the methods, the procedures, and the results of a scientific paper in direct and nonevaluative language. It is written not only to give a summary of the article, but also to attract the reader to the whole article. In manuscripts, abstracts are printed on a separate page. In printed articles, they are placed just before the introductory section begins.

According to the APA *Manual* (1994), a good abstract is accurate, self-contained, concise and specific, nonevaluative, and coherent and readable. The *Manual* limits the abstract of an empirical study to 960 characters and spaces. This approximates 120 words, but the student should count characters and spaces, not just words. Most computer word processors give an automatic count of the total number of characters and spaces in a document or its highlighted section. The *Manual* limits abstractions of theoretical articles to 75–100 words.

To conserve space, an abstract should be written in active voice. All numbers may be written in numerals instead of words. By recasting a sentence, the use of a number at its beginning is avoided.

Students often find it difficult to write an abstract of a paper. Writing an attractive and comprehensive abstract requires skills in precision writing. Exercises in abstracting a few papers are useful in learn-ing this skill.

An abstract, though brief, may have to be revised several times, especially if the first draft is too long. With a keen eye on wordiness, students can trim their abstracts to size.

Printed Notes	Class Notes

INTRODUCTION

The text of the paper starts with an introductory section without a heading. This section introduces: (1) the general area of investigation, (2) the general findings of past investigations, (3) the specific topic of the current investigation, (4) a review of selected studies that have dealt with the topic in the past, (5) the methods, results, conclusions, methodological problems, and limitations of the past studies, (6) the questions that remain to be answered, (7) the significance of the current investigation, and (8) the specific problem or research questions investigated in the present study.

The introduction should move from the general topic of investigation to the particular, specific research question investigated in the study. A critical review of previous studies sets the stage for the current investigation by pointing out gaps in our knowledge. This review should be fair, objective, and direct. The review should make clear to the reader the need for the study and the reasoning behind it. The review should show how the present study is related to past research while also pointing out its innovative aspects.

Toward the end of the introduction, the research question should be formally stated. Hypotheses, if proposed, may be stated at this point. The research questions and hypotheses must be written in direct, clear, and terse language. A good introduction gives sufficient background to the study and justifies its execution. By the end of this section, the reader should gain a clear understanding of the context of the study and why it was done.

Printed Notes	Class Notes

METHOD

The second section describes the method in detail for two reasons: (1) to give sufficient information to the reader who can understand the methods and procedures of the study to judge their appropriateness to investigate the research questions asked and (2) to permit direct and systematic replications of the study.

The method section consists of at least three subsections: (1) the subjects or participants, (2) the apparatus or materials, and (3) the procedure. Such additional subsections (and subheadings), as baselines or *Experiment 1, Experiment 2*, may be necessary.

Do not confuse the *Method* with *Procedures*. **Method** is a first level heading and **Procedures** is a second level heading.

Subjects (Participants)

The relevant characteristics of the participants (gender, age, education, cultural background, occupation, family background, health, geographical location, and communicative behaviors) are described. The number of participants and how they were selected also are specified in this subsection.

In clinical studies, the participants' diseases and disorders should be described in both qualitative and quantitative terms. Generally, any subject characteristic thought to influence the results should be described.

It is helpful to describe, when appropriate, the ethnocultural background of participants in a study. It is preferable to identify an ethnocultural group in the most precise terms possible. For example, instead of simply describing participants as *Asian Americans*, it may be helpful to specify, for example, that *20 Vietna-*

Printed Notes	Class Notes

mese and 20 Japanese American women participated in the study. Such specificity helps determine the generality of reported findings.

Materials

This subsection describes the physical setting of the study and the names and model numbers of equipment used. Such routine equipment as furniture may simply be mentioned, but description of any scientific or electronic instrument used should contain the name of the manufacturer and the model number. Instruments the investigator fabricates should be described in greater detail.

Standardized or nonstandardized tests and other assessment or rating procedures should be summarized. Photographs, diagrams, or additional descriptions may be included in an appendix if the apparatus is unusual or rarely used.

Procedures

This subsection describes in detail how the study was implemented. The experimental design should be identified and explained in detail if uncommon. The author should describe all stimuli presented to the subjects (including instructions given), how variables were measured and manipulated, and the temporal sequence of various conditions arranged in the study.

Differences in the treatment of groups of subjects should be explained, as well as reliability of the data. In reporting clinical treatment studies, the author should describe in detail the treatment procedures and how they were implemented. The methods by which the treatment ef-

Printed Notes	Class Notes

fects were measured and evaluated also should be described.

Other procedural information may be included in this section. In making this section complete, the author should follow the rule of providing all information necessary to replicate the study.

RESULTS

The results section opens with a brief statement of the problem investigated and the general findings of the study. An overview of the results is followed by a detailed presentation of quantitative, qualitative, graphic, and tabular presentation of the findings. These findings are reported without evaluations and interpretations.

Tables and graphs may be used to display data, and to supplement, not duplicate the text. Statistical or other procedures of data analysis should be specified and, when necessary, justified.

In organizing the results of a study, the student must consult the APA *Manual* and several exemplary articles published in the professional journal to which the author plans to submit the paper for publication.

DISCUSSION

In the discussion section, the author points out the meaning and significance of the results. This section is typically opened with a brief statement of the problem and the major findings. Discussion includes primarily the theoretical and applied implications of the findings. The current findings are related to those of previous investigations.

Limitations of the study also are pointed out, along with suggestions for further

Printed Notes	Class Notes

research. Ideally, a discussion is an integrative essay on the topic investigated, but it is written in light of the data generated by the study. It should answer the research questions posed in the introduction, as well as support or refute any hypotheses presented. Clarity and directness are important here. Excessive speculation on the causes of unexpected data should be avoided.

REFERENCES

The references section lists publications and other sources of information cited in the paper. The reference list should be accurate. It should be prepared according to an accepted format, such as that of the APA *Manual.* A reference list should list all of, and only, the sources cited in the paper.

Writing the Different Sections of a Research Paper

B.4.2. Write the *Review*, the *Methods*, and the *Results* of a Completed Study in the Past Tense

Incorrect	Correct
Deegook (1985) reports similar findings.	Deegook (1985) reported similar findings.
The author selects 10 male and 10 female subjects.	The author selected 10 male and 10 female subjects.
In assessing the hearing of the subjects, the Nicolet Aurora Model 1020 is used.	In assessing the hearing of the subjects, the Nicolet Aurora Model 1020 was used.
The results show that back massage is ineffective in reducing stuttering.	The results showed that back massage was ineffective in reducing stuttering.

B.4.3. Write the *Discussion* Section of a Completed Study in the Present Tense

Already completed study will have an extended discussion section. Research proposals may have a brief discussion section in which the meaning of expected results is suggested.

Incorrect	Correct
The data *suggested* that further research is needed.	The data *suggest* that further research is needed.
The observations *implied* that damage to Broca's area is unnecessary to produce Broca's aphasia.	The observations *imply* that damage to Broca's area is unnecessary to produce Broca's aphasia.

B.4.4. Write the *Review* Section of a Research Proposal in the Past Tense

Incorrect	Correct
The results of past studies show that patients with aphasia recover the most within the first 6 months of post-onset (Bikling, 1986; Thomas, 1992; Wise, 1988).	The results of past studies have shown that patients with aphasia recover the most within the first 6 months of post-onset (Bikling, 1986; Thomas, 1992; Wise).
Smith and Jones (1980) report that their test on central auditory processing is a useful diagnostic tool.	Smith and Jones (1980) reported that their test on central auditory processing is a useful diagnostic tool.

Writing the Different Sections of a Research Paper

B.4.2. Write the *Review*, the *Methods*, and the *Results* of a Completed Study in the Past Tense

Incorrect	Write Correctly
Smith (1989) believes that the classification of aphasia is an unnecessary exercise.	
Johnson (1967) uses the interview method to gather information on stuttering onset.	
The results of the Hanson (1988) study show that conductive hearing impairment is common in children.	

B.4.3. Write the *Discussion* Section of a Completed Study in the Present Tense

Incorrect	Write Correctly
The meaning of these results was not clear.	
The findings did not support the theory of unconscious control of the speech mechanism.	

B.4.4. Write the *Review* Section of a Research Proposal in the Past Tense

Incorrect	Write Correctly
The result of the Smith and Jones (1993) study supports the use of phonological analysis.	
Several past studies document the effectiveness of a well-designed aural rehabilitation program.	

B.4.5. Write the *Methods* and *Expected Results* Sections of a Research Proposal in the Future Tense

A proposal may have an **expected results** section in which the author describes the potential outcome of the proposed study.

Incorrect	Correct
I selected the subjects randomly.	I will select the subjects randomly. The subjects will be selected randomly.
I used the ABAB single-subject design.	I will use the ABAB single-subject design. The ABAB single-subject design will be used.
The results supported my hypothesis.	I expect the results to support my hypothesis.

B.4.5. Write the *Methods* and *Expected Results* Sections of a Proposal in the Future Tense

Incorrect	Write Correctly
I used 20 hearing impaired subjects in the study.	
I modeled when the client was unresponsive to my questions.	
The results suggested that cochlear implants were effective.	

Note to Students on Different Formats of Journal Articles

Besides research papers (articles), scientific and professional journals publish review papers, theoretical papers, tutorials, commentaries, and other kinds of papers. Each type of paper has an accepted format. Students should consult journals of their discipline and study types of papers and their prescribed formats.

PART C
PROFESSIONAL WRITING

INTRODUCTION TO PROFESSIONAL WRITING

Professional writing includes writing diagnostic or assessment reports, treatment plans, progress reports, and professional correspondence. As there is no standard accepted by all clinics, the names and the formats of these reports vary. However, many principles of good writing and those of scientific writing described in the previous sections of this book apply to professional writing as well. For example, rules of punctuation or those pertaining to quotations are applicable to clinical reports.

Certain aspects of the APA style may not be applicable to clinical reports. For example, clinical reports may vary from scientific reports in the size of margins, heading styles, indentations, and paragraph styles. The first line of the paragraph may or may not be indented. A significant deviation from the APA style is the common feature of one-sentence paragraphs in clinical reports. Because of a need for brevity, treatment targets, objectives, and various clinical criteria are often written in one-sentence paragraphs or even phrases (incomplete sentences). Clinical reports may contain recommendations written in the form of lists.

On the following pages, you will find examples of various clinical reports. I expect that the student clinicians and supervisors or instructors will use these as examples only; they are not meant to be prescriptive. Nonetheless, it is better for the beginning student to master a format than to enter the initial clinical practicum with no such format. An experienced clinician will have learned to vary the style to suit her or his employment setting and audience.

Clinicians in pubic schools, medical settings, and university clinics write vastly different kinds of reports. Reports vary not only in their formats, but also in the amount of details given. While some assessment reports are long enough to fill several pages, others are short enough to fill only a single page. Some contain connected prose, others contain only symbols, abbreviations, phrases, and brief observations. Generally, reports written in medical settings are briefer than those written in university speech and hearing clinics. Therefore, some student clinicians in university clinics ask why they are expected to write detailed reports that are uncommon in the "real world."

There are at least two good reasons for teaching student clinicians how to write reports with complete sentences and connected prose. First, even in settings that routinely require brief reports written with no complete sentences, there may be occasions when detailed, formal reports with extensive supportive evidence are required. When treatment has to be justified to a third party who pays for services or when a report comprehensible to other professionals has to be written, the clinician has to use a more narrative, cogent, and well-organized style. Second, the one who knows how to write a detailed report should have very little trouble writing brief reports. But the clinician that has learned only a brief and disconnected style will have great difficulty in writing elaborate, well-reasoned, well-organized narrative reports when such are needed.

The student clinicians should study the examples carefully and compare them with those written in their clinic. A simple rule of clinical practicum is to follow the guidelines of the setting in which that experience is offered. Therefore, it is the student clinicians' responsibility to find out what is acceptable in their setting.

consider your audience

C.1. DIAGNOSTIC REPORTS

Diagnostic reports also may be known as assessment reports and evaluation reports. In this book, the terms *diagnostic reports*, *assessment reports*, and *evaluation reports* are used interchangeably. Choose the term that is used in your setting.

ELEMENTS OF A DIAGNOSTIC REPORT

Although the formats vary, all diagnostic reports contain the following kinds of information:

- History of the client, the family, and the disorder
- Interview of the family, the client, or both
- Orofacial examination
- Hearing screening
- Speech and language samples
- Disorder-specific assessment including standardized and client-specific assessment procedures
- Diagnostic summary
- Recommendations

On the following pages, you will see outlines of typical diagnostic or assessment reports. Note that:

- The various headings and subheadings may vary across clinics and clinicians
- Most clinicians include information of the kind the headings suggest
- All headings and subheadings are not needed for all clients

---

C.1.1. OUTLINE OF A TYPICAL DIAGNOSTIC REPORT ON A
CHILD CLIENT

University Speech and Hearing Clinic
Victorville, California

DIAGNOSTIC REPORT

CLIENT: BIRTHDATE:

ADDRESS: CLINIC FILE NUMBER:

CITY: DATE OF REPORT:

TELEPHONE NUMBER: DIAGNOSIS:

REFERRED BY: CLINICIAN:

BACKGROUND AND REASONS FOR REFERRAL

HISTORY

Birth and Development

Medical History

Family, Social, and Educational History

ASSESSMENT INFORMATION

Orofacial Examination

Hearing Screening

Speech Production and Intelligibility

Language Production and Comprehension

Fluency

Voice

Diagnostic Summary

RECOMMENDATIONS

Submitted by_____

        Thomas Jefferson, B.A.

        Student Clinician

Client's or Parents' Signature_____

Approved By_____

        Mary Lincoln, M.A., CCC-SLP

        Speech-Language Pathologist and Clinical Supervisor

C.1.2. OUTLINE OF A TYPICAL DIAGNOSTIC REPORT ON AN
ADULT CLIENT

University Speech and Hearing Clinic
Jefferson City, North Carolina

DIAGNOSTIC REPORT

CLIENT: BIRTHDATE:

ADDRESS: CLINIC FILE NUMBER:

CITY: DATE OF REPORT:

TELEPHONE NUMBER: DIAGNOSIS:

REFERRED BY: CLINICIAN:

BACKGROUND AND REASONS FOR REFERRAL

HISTORY

Medical History

Family and Social History

Educational and Occupational History

ASSESSMENT INFORMATION

Orofacial Examination

Hearing Screening

Speech Production and Intelligibility

Language Production and Comprehension

Fluency

Voice

DIAGNOSTIC SUMMARY

RECOMMENDATIONS

Submitted by_____
          June Ahmed, B.A.
          Student Clinician

Client's signature_____

Approved By_____
          April Summers, M.A., CCC-SLP
          Speech-Language Pathologist and Clinical Supervisor

---

C.1.3. ANATOMY OF AN ASSESSMENT REPORT

University Speech and Hearing Clinic
1479 Wide Avenue
Boomtown, CA 90909

DIAGNOSTIC REPORT

CLIENT: Lynda Pen

ADDRESS: 555 N. Cedar
#000

CITY: Fresno, CA 93726

BIRTHDATE: xx-xx-xx

CLINIC FILE NUMBER:
87003

DIAGNOSIS: Language and
Articulation Disorders

TELEPHONE NUMBER:
555-0634

REFERRED BY:

DATE OF REPORT: xx-xx-xx

CLINICIAN:

BACKGROUND AND REASONS FOR REFERRAL

On September 15, 1997, Lynda Pen, a 7-year-old female, was evaluated at the University Speech and Hearing Clinic. She was referred by Dr. James Osborne, a pediatrician. Lynda's delayed expressive speech was the reason for referral. Mrs. Susan Penn brought her daughter to the clinic and provided the case history information.

The name of the clinic. Typically centered; may be all caps or in upper and lower case; bold

The type of report

Identifying Information. Arrange as shown.

---

level 1 heading (L1H)

Indented (5 spaces) paragraphs. Describe when, who, and how old a person was and referred to which clinic and why.

HISTORY

	(L1H)

Prenatal and Birth History

Mrs. Pen reported that she experienced preeclampsia 5 months into her pregnancy. At 30 weeks of gestation, Lynda was delivered by a Cesarean section. Birthweight was 5 pounds and 8 ounces. Because of cardiac murmurs and a premature birth, Lynda did not thrive during her first 6 months of development.

Level 2 Heading (L2H)

Start with prenatal and birth history. Mother's health during pregnancy. Birth: normal or otherwise. Early development. Health during infancy and early childhood.

Developmental History

Lynda's developmental milestones were reported to be delayed for both physical and communicative behaviors. Mrs. Pen reported that Lynda walked at 26 months and "used a few single words" at 24 months. Mrs. Pen stated that currently, Lynda's speech consists of 10–15 word-approximations.

(L2H)

Describe later development and physical growth. Communicative behaviors. Current status.

Medical History

Mrs. Pen reported that Lynda had a single instance of otitis media at 9 months of age. At 10 months of age, Lynda underwent a specialized heart surgery called pulmonary banding to prevent further damage to her lungs. At 2 years of age, Lynda was operated on at the University of California Hospital in San Francisco by Drs. T. S. Musclemouster and O. S. Housterhouter for anterior skull reconstruction. At the age of 2 years and 2 months, Lynda underwent open-heart surgery to repair cardiac murmurs. The Medical Genetics Team at Valley Children's Hospital has reported that Lynda has a probable chromosome abnormality with extra material on chromosome 14q.

(L2H)

Summarize significant medical history, including sensory problems, medical and surgical treatment, and any previously made diagnostic statements.

Family, Social, and Educational History

Mrs. Pen does not recall any members of her family or those of her husband's as having speech or language problems. Lynda is the only child of Mr. and Mrs. Pen. Mr. Pen is a high school teacher, and Mrs. Pen is an insurance underwriter. Lynda's grandmother, who lives with Mr. and Mrs. Pen, usually watches her when the parents are at work.

Lynda sometimes plays with a younger child in the neighborhood. According to Mrs. Pen, Lynda generally plays cooperatively with children who are younger than she is.

(L2H)

Describe the family history of communicative problems. Describe the family. How many children? Patient's education and occupation. Who takes care of the child? Child's companions and play activities.

Lynda attended the clinic of Exceptional Parents Unlimited from May 1987 to April 1988. Mrs. Pen reported that Lynda interacted well with her peers although the frequency of her social interactions was limited. Lynda is not currently attending school.

ASSESSMENT INFORMATION

Orofacial Examination

An orofacial examination was conducted to evaluate the structural and functional integrity of the oral-facial mechanism. The examination revealed a broad nasal bridge and prominent epicanthal folds. The teeth were marked by a Class III malocclusion. During smiling, there was bilateral retraction at the angle of the mouth. A narrow, inverted v-shaped palate also was noted. Due to Lynda's lack of cooperation, movements of the velum and the lateral pharyngeal walls were not observed. Labial and lingual mobility was deemed adequate for normal speech production.

Speech Production and Intelligibility

Lynda's speech was assessed through a standardized test and a recorded conversational speech sample. To assess Lynda's speech production in fixed word positions, the Goldman-Fristoe Test of Articulation was administered. Her performance on this test revealed numerous errors of articulation as summarized in the following table.

	Initial	Medial	Final
Substitutions	t/s; d/p	s/z	
	d/dr; k/kr; p/pl; s/sl; t/tr		

Sidebar annotations:

Describe the previous clinical and education program of relevance and the current educational level.

(L1H)

(L2H)

Describe the orofacial examination: Integrity of oral and facial structures. Give a general description of the face, mouth, tongue, teeth, hard and soft palate, and movement of the soft palate and the tongue.

(L2H)

First, say how speech production was assessed. Give the full name of tests administered. Do not ignore speech samples.

List errors of articulation noted on the test or tests administered.

Arrange the errors of articulation in a table as shown.

Omissions	/f, v, t, n, s, z, l, r, w, h, fl, st/	/b, m, f, d, n, s, l, r/	/p, b, m, f, v, t, n, s, r, k/
Distortions	/s/		

A 90-utterance speech sample was tape recorded. An analysis of this sample revealed the following additional errors:

	Initial	Medial	Final
Substitutions	p/b; b/m; t/s; y/l		
Omissions	/m, k/ ts; fl	/g/	/d, l, k/ ts
Distortions	/z, s/		

Because of her numerous errors of articulation, Lynda's speech was generally unintelligible. With contextual cues present, her speech intelligibility was only 11.9% on a word-by-word and an utterance-by-utterance basis.

Language Production and Comprehension

Lynda's language production was assessed mainly through a language sample. She responded to questions and was asked to describe pictures in storybooks. Through this method, a 90-utterance language sample was obtained. An analysis of this sample showed a Mean Length of Utterance (MLU) of 1.13 for words. She did not produce any syntactically complete sentences as she said mostly one-word phrases. Because of reduced speech intelligibility marked by sound substitutions and omissions, Lynda's use of morphologic features could not be assessed.

Lynda's comprehension of words was assessed by administering the Assessment of Children's Language Comprehension (ACLC). The following results were obtained: Part A: 76%; Part B: 80%; Part C: 10%; and Part D: 20%. These results suggest that her comprehension of words is poor.

Describe the speech sample. List the errors of articulation noted in the speech sample.

Arrange the errors of articulation in a table like this.

Describe the effects of articulation errors on intelligibility.

(L2H)

Describe how you assessed language production. Give names of tests you administered. Describe the method of analysis. Describe the results of analysis. Describe limitations (something not done).

Describe how you assessed comprehension. Describe the results.

Voice and Fluency

Based on the clinical observations, Lynda's vocal pitch and intensity were judged appropriate for her age. Because of her limited speech and language production, Lynda's fluency also was limited. However, clinically significant amounts or durations of dysfluencies were not observed.

DIAGNOSTIC SUMMARY

The overall results of the assessment of Lynda Pen's speech and language production show severe articulation and expressive language difficulties. Lynda's speech was characterized by reduced intelligibility due to many omitted and substituted phonemes and inconsistent production of others. Expressive language was limited mostly to one-word utterances. This resulted in limited fluency although her vocal characteristics were within the limits of normal variations. The assessment results also suggest that Lynda's comprehension of language was limited.

(L2H)

Comment on voice and fluency.

Say your judgments were based on speech sample or samples.

(L1H)

Summarize the communicative problems noted in the assessment.

Highlight the major problems that may be the targets for immediate intervention.

RECOMMENDATIONS

It is recommended that Lynda Pen receive treatment for her speech and language problems. Among others to be determined later, the treatment targets may include the following:

1. Spontaneous naming of pictures of her family members with 90% accuracy.
2. Spontaneous naming of selected, functional words with 90% accuracy.
3. Production of phrases and sentences in a carefully graded sequence.
4. Correct production of selected phonemes.

Submitted by_____

    LaTeena LeBueque, B.A.
    Student Clinician

Parent's signature_____

    Mrs. Susan Penn

Approved By_____

    Benton Q. Bentley, M.A., CCC-SLP
    Speech-Language Pathologist and
    Clinical Supervisor

(L1H)

Do you recommend treatment? What are some of the priority treatment targets?

List the potential targets as shown.

List as many targets as seem appropriate.

Name and signature of the student clinician

Parent's signature

Signature and name, degree, ASHA certificate, and title of the supervisor

Note to Student Clinicians

Use the preceding anatomy of an assessment report to understand the general content of a report. Consult your clinic's format for writing assessment reports. The format may vary, but the essential content is likely to be substantially similar to what is presented in the report.

C.1.4. SAMPLE DIAGNOSTIC REPORTS

Note to Student Clinicians

On the following pages, you will see samples of diagnostic (assessment) reports. Study them for the general content and format of diagnostic reports. Compare the samples with the format used in your clinic. Take note of variations in headings and their styles used in your clinic. Consult with your clinic director or clinical supervisor to select an approved format and acceptable variations, if any.

C.1.4. SAMPLE DIAGNOSTIC REPORT: *ARTICULATION DISORDER*

University Speech and Hearing Clinic
Midstate University
Middletown, Montana

DIAGNOSTIC REPORT

CLIENT: Pennifer Forbes

ADDRESS: 1326 E. Harvard

CITY: Middletown, Montana

TELEPHONE NUMBER: 555-0719

REFERRED BY: Jane Pendelton, M.D.

BIRTHDATE: xx-xx-xx

CLINIC FILE NUMBER: 9-QR101

DATE OF REPORT: xx-xx-xx

DIAGNOSIS: Articulation/Phonological Disorder

CLINICIAN: Missouline Montoya

BACKGROUND AND REASONS FOR REFERRAL

Pennifer Forbes, a 5-year-old female, was seen on February x, xxxx for an evaluation at the Speech and Hearing Clinic at the Midstate University, Middletown, Montana. Dr. Pendelton, a pediatrician, referred her to the clinic because of her articulation problems. Pennifer was accompanied to the clinic by her mother, Mrs. Jane Forbes, who served as the informant.

HISTORY

Mrs. Forbes reported that Pennifer's speech is difficult to understand. She said that her daughter leaves out sounds in her speech resulting in such words as "nake" for "snake." Pennifer also substitutes one sound for another. According to the mother, Pennifer says, "tat" for "cat." Pennifer has previously received speech therapy at Big Sky Speech and Hearing Center for remediation of her articulation disorder. The 3-month treatment she received resulted in some improvement, but Pennifer's speech problems are still significant.

Pennifer's birth and developmental history is not remarkable. Her motor and speech development was typical as judged by Mrs. Forbes. Pennifer has enjoyed good health with no diseases of significance.

Family, Social, and Educational History

Pennifer is the second of three children. Mrs. Forbes did not report a family history of communicative disorders. Mrs. Forbes, a high school graduate, manages a restaurant. Mr. Forbes, who did not finish high school education, is a maintenance man with the local school district.

Pennifer attends a kindergarten school and is reportedly doing well. However, other students and the teacher have complained about her unintelligible speech.

Oral-Peripheral Examination

An oral-peripheral examination was performed to assess the function and integrity of the oral mechanism. Pennifer's lips and hard palate appeared symmetrical at rest. She was able to perform a variety of labial and lingual tasks. The anterior and posterior faucial pillars were within normal limits. Vertical movement of the pharyngeal wall was observed upon the phonation of /a/.

Hearing Screening

Using a Maico portable screening audiometer (model MA-20A), the clinician screened Pennifer's hearing at 25 dB HL for 250, 500, 1000, 2000, 4000, and 8000 Hz. At all frequencies, Pennifer passed the screening bilaterally.

Speech Production and Intelligibility

To assess Pennifer's speech sound production, a conversational speech sample was recorded. In addition, the Goldman Fristoe Test of Articulation (GFTA) was administered to assess speech sounds in fixed positions. An analysis of the speech sample and Pennifer's performance on the GFTA revealed the following errors:

	Initial	Medial	Final
Substitutions	/s/ for /k/; /d/ for /g/ /t/ for /s/; /w/ for /r/ /b/ for /f/; /t/ for /ch/ /t/ for /sh/, /j/ for /z/ /b/ for /bl/, /b/ for /br/, /d/ for /dr/, /bl/ for /fl/, /t/ for /kl/, /l/ for /sl/, /d/ for /st/	/l/ for /t/; /t/ for /sh/; /b/ for /v/; /d/ for /g/; /b/ for /f/; /t/ for /ch/	/k/ for /t/
Omissions		/k/ /th/	/g/, /k/, /d/, /f/, /s/, /t/, /sh/, /ch/, /th/ (unvoiced), /l/, /d/, /z/, /p/
Distortions		/z/	

The Khan-Lewis Phonological Analysis was administered to assess Pennifer's phonological error patterns. Pennifer's overall score of 32 on the test was calculated into an age equivalency of 2 to 9 years. The analysis revealed the following phonological processes:

Deletion of final consonants

Initial voicing

Palatal fronting

Velar fronting

Stridency deletion

Stopping of affricates and fricatives

Cluster simplification

Final devoicing

Liquid simplification

Due to numerous errors of articulation, only 23% of Pennifer's sentences were intelligible. In addition, most of her misarticulations were not stimulable. Pennifer correctly imitated only /k/, /g/, /s/, and /f/. However, a diadochokinetic test showed essentially normal rates.

Language Production and Comprehension

Pennifer's conversational speech during the interview and assessment showed essentially normal language structure and use except for several missing grammatical morphemes. It is possible that missing grammatical morphemes are due to missing speech sounds. The mean length of utterance (MLU) of her speech sample was 5.4 morphemes, which is within normal limits for her age.

Voice and Fluency

Though difficult to understand, Pennifer's speech had normal rhythm. The rate of dysfluencies was within the normal range. Therefore, no further analysis of the dysfluency rate was made. In addition, Pennifer's voice was judged to be within normal limits.

DIAGNOSTIC SUMMARY

Pennifer Forbes exhibits a severe articulation disorder characterized by multiple misarticulations and limited speech intelligibility. Unless treated, her articulation disorder is likely to have negative social and educational consequences. Because Pennifer was stimulable for some of the consonants, the prognosis for improvement is good.

RECOMMENDATIONS

It is recommended that Pennifer receive treatment for her articulation disorder. As articulation and intelligibility improves, Pennifer's language may be further evaluated to see if morphological features emerge. If they do not, language treatment should be offered.

Submitted by_____

       Missouline Montoya, B.A.
       Student Clinician

Parent's signature_____

       Mrs. Jane Forbes

Approved By_____

       Akbar Jamal, M.A., CCC-SLP
       Speech-Language Pathologist
       Clinical Supervisor

C.1.4. SAMPLE DIAGNOSTIC REPORT: *VOICE DISORDER*

Balmtown University Speech and Hearing Clinic
Balmtown, New York

DIAGNOSTIC REPORT

NAME: VALINE WRENN

BIRTHDATE: xx-xx-xx

AGE: 25

ADDRESS: 1919 S. Dakota #Q108-R

CITY: Fresno, CA 98705

TELEPHONE: 555-0608

DATE OF EXAMINATION: xx-xx-xx

CLINICAL CLASSIFICATION: VOICE DISORDER

CLINIC FILE NO: 08A-7314

REFERRED BY: DR. HANNA EISMER

EXAMINER: JANINA PRESHAM

INFORMANT: SELF

BACKGROUND AND PRESENTING COMPLAINTS

Valine Wrenn, a 25-year-old female, was seen for a speech and language evaluation at the Balmtown University Speech and Hearing Clinic on April xx, xxxx. She was referred to the clinic by her otolaryngologist, Dr. Eismer. Her presenting complaints were difficulty speaking loudly and difficulty speaking for long periods. She also noted a "lack of excitement" in her voice and difficulty producing sounds at the ends of sentences due to a low pitch. Valine came to the Clinic by herself and provided all the information.

HISTORY

Early History

Valine reported that her voice always sounded "funny" since early childhood. During her high school years, she became aware of a low pitch and monotone quality after listening to herself on audiotape. Valine did not recall previous consultations or treatment for her voice problem. She thought that her developmental history was unremarkable.

Medical History

On March xx, xxxx, Valine received a medical evaluation by Dr. Hanna Eismer, an otolaryngologist. Dr. Eismer reported Valine as having normal external auditory canals and tympanic membranes. The nose and oral cavities were also clear. A fiberoptic endoscope was used to examine Valine's larynx. Vocal fold structure and motion were reported to be normal. There was no evidence of vocal nodules or lesions. The vocal folds were described as being minimally erythematous (redness of tissue) and slightly swollen on the free edge.

Valine reported having allergies to molds, trees, and grasses. These affected her only when she was in close proximity to one of them, causing excessive phlegm in the throat and postnasal drip. Valine recently began using Beconase (an inhalant) to relieve the allergies. Valine also had excessive colds resulting in phlegm and postnasal drip. These were noted as occurring approximately once a month beginning in October or November, and lasting about a week. Valine thought that her colds were caused by stress and emotional problems. She temporarily discontinued the use of the Beconase while using Afrin and Neo-Synephrine for the colds. Excessive phlegm resulted in frequent coughing and throat clearing.

Family, Social, and Educational History

Valine is a student at the Balmtown University, Balmtown, New York, majoring in speech communication. She is divorced and lives with her 3-year-old daughter, Haline. Either the television or the radio is on in Valine's apartment for the majority of the time she is at home. While speaking to her daughter, Valine rarely shouts or yells through the apartment. Instead, she makes an effort to go into the room where her daughter is. Valine noted that she frequently sings for personal pleasure. She sings in numerous and varied settings, including at home, in the car, and on campus. She has between 2–5 telephone conversations per day, ranging from 2 to 30 minutes in length. Valine does not habitually drink coffee, tea, soft drinks, or alcoholic beverages. She does drink at least two glasses of low-fat milk every day. Valine mentioned that friends easily identify her voice and describe it as being "low and sexy." Valine typically experiences a feeling of tightness in the throat when nervous, as well as a higher pitch, lower intensity, and difficulty projecting her voice.

ASSESSMENT INFORMATION

Orofacial Examination

An orofacial examination was conducted to assess the integrity of oral and facial structures. Valine's facial features appeared symmetrical, with lingual and labial mobility adequate for speech. However, restricted oral mobility was noted during speech. Velopharyngeal closure was acoustically deemed adequate during repeated productions of /a/. Diadochokinetic rates were within normal limits.

Hearing Screening

Using a Maico portable screening audiometer (model MA-20A), the clinician screened Valine's hearing at 25 dB HL for 250, 500, 1000, 2000, 4000, and 8000 Hz. At all frequencies, Valine passed the screening bilaterally.

Speech Production and Comprehension

Valine's speech production and comprehension were informally assessed. Her conversational speech and her interaction during the interview did not reveal speech production or comprehension problems. Therefore, these aspects of her communicative behaviors were judged to be within normal variations.

Language and Fluency

Valine's language and fluency were assessed informally. Her conversational speech during the assessment period did not suggest problems of language structure or use. Her fluency and rates of dysfluencies also were judged to be within normal variations.

Voice

Valine's fundamental frequency ranged between 150 Hz and 200 Hz on the fundamental frequency indicator. This pitch was determined to be low for Valine's gender and stature. During the interview, frequent glottal fry and hoarseness of voice were observed. A later analysis of the audiotaped speech sample revealed that glottal fry and hoarseness were more likely to occur on downward inflections of most utterances. On approximately 60% of her utterances, either glottal fry, hoarseness, or both were observed. However, Valine's breath support appeared adequate for speech.

DIAGNOSTIC SUMMARY

Valine Wrenn's history suggests vocally abusive behaviors. She uses a habitual pitch that is too low for her. This may have resulted in excessive glottal fry. She also used a low vocal focus, which may have adversely affected the extent to which she could project her voice.

RECOMMENDATIONS

It was recommended that Valine Wrenn receive voice therapy. Specific recommendations include:

1. Eliminating glottal fry by raising Valine's habitual pitch to a more optimal level during spontaneous conversational speech produced in nonclinical settings.

2. Decreasing such abusive vocal behaviors as ineffective management of colds and allergies, improper fluid intake, and singing and speaking in noisy situations.

Submitted by_____

            Janina Presham, B.A.
            Student Clinician

Client's signature_____

            Valine Wrenn

Approved By_____

            Dambly Doumbleson, M.A., CCC-SLP
            Clinical Supervisor and Speech-Language Pathologist

---

C.1.4. SAMPLE DIAGNOSTIC REPORT: *APHASIA AND APRAXIA*

University Speech and Hearing Clinic
Tinkyville, Tennessee

DIAGNOSTIC REPORT

NAME: Lynn M. Zoolanfoos

BIRTHDATE: xx-xx-xx

ADDRESS: 111 E. Cornell

CLINIC FILE NUMBER: 910019

CITY: Tinkyville, TN 43704

DIAGNOSIS: Aphasia and Apraxia

TELEPHONE NUMBER: 677-229-9850

DATE OF REPORT: xx-xx-xx

CLINICIAN: Maxine Traoumer

SUPERVISOR: Galaxy Galvestrouton, M.A., CCC-SLP

REFERRED BY: Dr. Mendelsohn

ASSESSMENT DATE: xx-xx-xx

BACKGROUND AND REASONS FOR REFERRAL

Lynn Zoolanfoos, a 44-year-old female, was referred to the Speech and Hearing Clinic at the Tinkyville State University in Tinkyville, Tennessee. Her physician, Dr. Muskwhiter Mendelsohn referred her for a speech-language evaluation following a stroke.

Lynn's speech and language were evaluated in two sessions. She was seen on September xx, xxxx and October xx, xxxx. Lynn was unaccompanied to the diagnostic sessions. She suffered an initial stroke in July of xxxx. On September xx, xxxx, she experienced a second stroke which resulted in right hemiplegia, expressive and receptive aphasia, and verbal apraxia.

HISTORY

Medical History

Lynn has a history of heart problems. She resides with her mother, Gladys Miller, who experiences severe emphysema and is on continuous oxygen. Lynn and her mother have a home care aide who comes into the home 6 hours a day.

Lynn reported she wears braces on her right leg and right hand and uses a cane to assist with walking. Lynn enjoys activities such as bowling and watching television. She now wants to improve her writing skills.

Previous Speech and Language Services

For the past 6 months, Lynn has received speech and language services at the Community Hospital Speech and Hearing Department. Previous treatment targets include the production of two-to-four-word phrases; correct production of initial and final consonants in single words; auditory comprehension of two-and-three-step directions and two-and-three-element questions; and reading comprehension of three-to-six-word sentences.

ASSESSMENT INFORMATION

Lynn cooperated during the evaluation and showed excellent motivation for continuing therapy. She was keenly interested in the assessment tasks. She said that she wanted to improve her speech and language skills.

Orofacial Examination

An orofacial examination was performed to evaluate the functional and structural integrity of the oral-facial complex. Facial features including lips at rest were judged symmetrical and normal in appearance and function. The tongue was normal in appearance, but its lateral movements were sluggish. There were groping behaviors while attempting to draw the tip of the tongue along the hard palate. A slight neutroclusion was noted. The hard palate was narrow, with a high arch and a small bony outgrowth along the midline. Pronounced rugae were evident in the premaxillary region. The soft palate was of adequate length and elevated vertically and posteriorly to achieve closure. Velopharyngeal functioning was acoustically judged to be adequate during production of /a/. An assessment of diadochokinetic rates revealed slowness suggesting weakness in circumoral and lingual musculature. The productions also were characterized by substitutions suggesting verbal apraxia.

Voice

Lynn's voice characteristics were subjectively judged based on her conversational speech. Except for a hyponasal resonance, her voice was judged appropriate for her age and gender.

Hearing Screening

A hearing screening was performed bilaterally at 25 dB HL for 250, 500, 1000, 2000, 4000, and 8000 Hz. Lynn passed at all frequencies bilaterally.

Speech Production

The Apraxia Battery for Adults was administered to verify the presence of apraxia and provide a rough estimate of the severity of the disorder. The summary of scores were as follows:

Subtest I	Diadochokinetic Rate
p t	13
t k	10
p t k	6

Subtest II	Increasing Word Length
1 syllable average	1.8
2 syllable average	1.7
3 syllable average	1.9
Deterioration in performance score	0

Subtest III	Limb Apraxia and Oral Apraxia
Limb Apraxia	34
Oral Apraxia	39

Subtest IV	Latency and Utterance Time for Polysyllabic Words
Latency Time	93 seconds
Utterance Time	2 seconds
	Repeated Trials Test

Subtest V	
Total Amount of Change	+1
Subtest VI	Inventory of Articulation Characteristics of Apraxia
Total YES Items	2

Lynn's performance on the subtests reveals searching behaviors for making gestures and a low score on articulation characteristics of apraxia.

Language Production and Comprehension

A 76-utterance, 157-word language sample was obtained. The Mean-Length-of-Utterance for these utterances was 2.19 for words and 2.42 for morphemes. Word finding difficulties were noted. Automatic speech was evident in some of her replies.

To make an initial assessment of Lynn's aphasia, the first three items of each subtest of the Western Aphasia Battery were administered as a screening test. In the following table, Lynn's scores are listed in the left-hand column. Several subtests were scored beyond the first three items. These scores are listed in the right-hand column. The scores were as follows:

	Client's Subscores on first three items/Maximum	Client's Subscores beyond the first three items/Maximum
Spontaneous Speech		
Information Content	6/10	
Fluency	5/10	
Yes/No Questions	9/9	36/42
Auditory Word Recognition	9/27	
Sequential Commands	6/6	8/22
Repetition	6/6	60/70
Word Fluency	2/20	
Sentence Completion	4/6	6/10
Responsive Speech	0/6	
Reading	20.5/32	30.5/52
Writing	31.5/100	
Praxis	6/6	27/30
Drawing	3/9	
Calculation	0/4	

Lynn performed well on tasks involving auditory comprehension for yes/no questions, auditory comprehension of one-part sequential commands, verbal repetition of single words and two-to-five-word phrases, sentence completion, and reading single words. Errors were noted during tasks involving oral reading of phrases and sentences, spelling, writing (except for writing numbers and her own name and copying printed words), calculation, drawing, responsive speech, word fluency, auditory word recognition, spontaneous speech, and two-part sequential commands. Lynn's performance on the Praxis subtest did not suggest oral or verbal apraxia. An Aphasia Quotient and a Cortical Quotient were unobtainable due to partial presentation of the test.

DIAGNOSTIC SUMMARY

Lynn's performance on various assessment tasks suggests a moderate to severe expressive and receptive aphasia with anomia. A mild verbal apraxia is also suggested.

RECOMMENDATIONS

Speech and language treatment is recommended for Lynn. Immediate treatment goals recommended for her include the following:

1. Improve expressive language.
2. Teach consistent productions of selected functional words and phrases. These productions may include a variety of communication modes (gesturing, drawing, speaking, writing) to improve communicative effectiveness.

3. Teach four-to-six-word sentence completion performance with 90% accuracy.
4. Improve receptive language in reading.
5. Teach correct responses to questions about silently read material with 90% accuracy.

Submitted by_____
        Maxine Traoumer, B.A.
        Student Clinician

Client's signature_____
        Lynn Zoolanfoos

Approved By_____
        Galaxy Galvestrouton, M.A., CCC-SLP
        Speech-Language Pathologist and Clinical Supervisor

C.1.4. SAMPLE DIAGNOSTIC REPORT: *STUTTERING*

University Speech and Hearing Clinic
Freemont University
Valleyville, California

DIAGNOSTIC REPORT

NAME: James Foxx   ASSESSMENT DATE: xx-xx-xx

BIRTHDATE: xx-xx-xx   FILE NUMBER: RS92019

ADDRESS: Graves 312 B   DIAGNOSIS: Stuttering

CITY: Valleyville, CA 90710-3342   DATE OF REPORT: xx-xx-xx

TELEPHONE NUMBER: 555-3235   INFORMANT: Self

REFERRED BY: SELF   CLINICIAN: Meena Wong

BACKGROUND AND PRESENTING COMPLAINT

James Foxx, a 21-year-old male, was seen for a speech and language evaluation at the Freemont University Speech and Hearing Clinic on February x, xxxx. He had applied for services for his stuttering after he read an article in the campus newspaper about the speech and hearing services on campus. James is a student at the university, majoring in computer science.

HISTORY

James reported that, according to what his parents have told him, his stuttering began when he was about 3 years of age. From the age of 4 through 9 years, James received treatment for his stuttering at J. R. Cronin Elementary School in Dublin, California. At age 7, he also received approximately a year of treatment at Motherlode University, Red Wing. He has not received treatment since that time. James reported that the severity of his stuttering fluctuates depending on his mood, and it is more pronounced in stressful situations.

He reports increased frequency of stuttering when he speaks to strangers, his instructors, and his father. He thinks he is less dysfluent when he speaks to his mother, brother, sister, and close friends. He said that he would rather not order at restaurants, buy tickets at counters, introduce himself, or answer telephone calls. He does not think that he has difficulty with specific words or sounds.

Family and Social History

James lives on campus. His parents live in Merced, California. He is the oldest of three children. His younger brother and younger sister do not have communication problems. He believes that his maternal uncle and his son both stutter. James is not aware of any person on his father's side who stutters.

James lives with a roommate in a dorm on the campus. He says that his verbal interactions with his roommate are limited. He has other friends with whom he spends more time. Reportedly, he has difficulty asking for dates because he is worried that he might stutter badly.

Educational and Occupational History

James had part-time jobs in various businesses. He believes that his stuttering was always a frustrating problem in the work place. He usually avoided speaking to his supervisors. He tended to seek work that did not involve much oral communication.

James is studying for a degree in computer science. He is doing well in his courses. He does not think that his stuttering has negatively affected his coursework or relationship with his instructors. He plans to work for a private company when he finishes his degree. He is concerned about being able to communicate under job pressure. James appears to be highly motivated for treatment, as he wants to be able to speak fluently.

ASSESSMENT INFORMATION

Orofacial Examination

An orofacial examination was performed to assess the structural and functional integrity of the oral mechanism. The examination did not reveal anything of clinical significance.

Types and Frequency of Dysfluencies

To analyze the types and the frequency of dysfluencies, a conversational speech sample was recorded. James was also asked to bring an audiotaped conversational speech sample within the next 3 days. An analysis of the two samples revealed the following types and frequency of dysfluencies.

Dysfluency Types	Clinic Sample Total Words: 1231		Home Sample Total Words: 1071
	Frequency of Dysfluency	% of Total Dysfluency	Frequency of Dysfluency
Interjections	86	6.9	26
Pauses	29	2.3	9
Part-word reps	68	5.5	60
Whole-word reps	9	7	57
Audible prolongations	52	4.2	4
Silent prolongations	7	0.6	4
Revisions	8	6	6
Incomplete phrases	2	0.2	1
TOTAL	**261**		**199**
PERCENT DYS. RATE	**21**		**18.6**

Both the speech samples contained pauses from 5–25 seconds in duration. His sound and silent prolongations typically exceeded 1 sec. James's rate of speech was calculated between 110 and 150 words per minute depending on the amount and duration of pauses and prolongations. He intermittently rushed groups of words. Overall rate of speech was variable depending on amount of dysfluencies.

An occasional eye blink and hand movements associated with dysfluencies were observed during the interview. These motor behaviors were most often associated with part-word repetitions and silent and sound prolongations.

Language Production and Comprehension

An informal assessment of a 100-utterance, 1,231-word, conversational language sample revealed expressive language skills that were judged appropriate for his level of education. No language comprehension problems were noted during the interview.

Voice

James spoke with laryngeal tension and hard glottal attack approximately 50% of the time. Tension and abrupt initiation of voice were often associated with dysfluencies. Nonetheless, he exhibited appropriate vocal intensity, intonation, and inflectional patterns.

Hearing Screening

A bilateral hearing screening was administered at 25 dB HL for 250, 500, 1000, 2000, 4000, 6000, and 8000 Hz. James responded to all frequencies.

DIAGNOSTIC SUMMARY

Analysis of the conversational speech samples revealed that James Foxx exhibits a severe fluency disorder with 18 to 21% dysfluency rates. His dominant dysfluencies are repetitions, prolongations, interjections, and pauses.

RECOMMENDATIONS

It is recommended that James Foxx receive treatment for his stuttering in which the following fluency skills be taught within a fluency-shaping program:

1. Teaching appropriate airflow, rate reduction, and gentle phonatory onset.
2. Production of 98% fluent speech within the clinic.
3. Maintenance of at least 95% fluency in extraclinical situations.

Submitted by_____
        Meena Wong, B.A.
        Student Clinician

Client's signature_____
        James Foxx

Approved By_____
        Nancy Lopez, M.A., CCC-SLP
        Speech-Language Pathologist and Clinical Supervisor

C.I.5. PRACTICE IN CLINICAL REPORT WRITING

Note to Student Clinicians

In practicing diagnostic report writing in the next section, use the information given on the left-hand pages and write your report on the right-hand pages. Give appropriate headings and subheadings. Invent missing information.

Take note that the information on the left-hand pages is often written in an abbreviated style. You should not simply copy these truncated constructions. You should use the information to write formal, well-connected, reports.

C.1.5. ASSESSMENT REPORT: *ARTICULATION DISORDER*

Data Sheet. Use these data to write your report on the opposite page. Use the correct headings.

Name of the clinic, city, and state: (invent)

| Write the name and address of the clinic |

DIAGNOSTIC REPORT

What kind of report? **(L1H)**

Mathew Moon, client; age, 8; address: (invent) telephone: (invent); clinician: yourself; date of assessment: (invent); diagnosis: articulation disorder; referred by Dr. Lydia Bong, a counselor.

Identifying information Arrange appropriately

BACKGROUND AND REASONS FOR REFERRAL

(L1H)

Use the information above
No prior assessment
Informant: Mr. Sonny Moon, father
Date seen and evaluated (invent)

Who, how old a person, referred when, to which clinic, and why?

Write your report. Use the information on the data sheet. Invent information as needed.

Data Sheet. Use these data to write your report on the opposite page. Use the correct headings.

HISTORY

(L1H)

Birth and Development

(L2H)

Normal pregnancy, Cesarean delivery

No other prenatal or natal complications

Normal infancy

Delayed motor development, but no specific information

First words at 18 months

Soon language development somewhat accelerated to approximate the normal

Prenatal, birth
Mother's health
Early development

Early language development

Medical History

(L2H)

Frequent middle ear infections; frequent medical treatment

Mild conductive hearing loss according to previous clinical reports

Frequent attacks of cold and allergies

Chicken pox at 4

Diseases of significance

Write your report. Use the information on the data sheet. Invent information as needed.

_____

_____

_____

_____

_____

_____

_____

_____

_____

_____

_____

_____

_____

_____

_____

_____

_____

_____

_____

_____

_____

_____

_____

_____

_____

_____

_____

_____

Data Sheet. Use these data to write your report on the opposite page. Use the correct headings.	
Family, Social, and Educational History	**(L2H)**
An older brother (10 years), a younger sister (2 years)	Family How many children?
None with a communicative disorder	Any family history of communicative problems?
Mother: college graduate; a real estate broker Father: high school graduate; car repairman	Parent's education and occupation
Mathew, in 2nd grade, doing below average school work, was held back the first year in school	Educational information
He plays well with other children Parents say he is cooperative, affectionate, and well behaved Gets group speech treatment at his school once a week for 20 minutes	Child's companions and social behavior Any other information about the family

Write your report. Use the information on the data sheet. Invent information as needed.

Data Sheet. Use these data to write your report on the opposite page. Use the correct headings.

ASSESSMENT INFORMATION

(L1H)

Orofacial Examination

(L2H)

Class II malocclusion

Sluggish lingual movements

No other findings of significance

Describe the orofacial examination: integrity of oral and facial structures.

Give a general description of the face, mouth, teeth, tongue, hard and soft palate, and movement of the soft palate and the tongue.

Hearing Screening

(L2H)

Screened: 250, 500, 1000, 2000, 4000, and 8000 Hz at 25 dB HL

Failed at all tested frequencies

Needs a complete audiological examination; will be referred to an audiologist

What frequencies were screened and at what level?

What were the results?

Write your report. Use the information on the data sheet. Invent information as needed.

Data Sheet. Use these data to write your report on the opposite page. Use the correct headings.

Speech Production and Intelligibility

Conversational speech sample

Goldman-Fristoe Test of Articulation

Numerous errors in both

In the initial position of words, omitted: /b, d, p, f, v, r, k/; substituted: t/k; distorted: /z, s/

In the medial position of words, omitted: /b, m, f, z, s, l, g, r/

In the final position of words, omitted: /b, d, p, f, v, r, k, t, l, m, n, s/

The same errors in conversational speech

Intelligibility with contextual cues: 75% for utterances

(L2H)

How was speech production assessed?

Give the full name of tests administered. Do not ignore speech samples.

Summarize the errors in a table.

What was the speech intelligibility?

Write your report. Use the information on the data sheet. Invent information as needed.

_____

_____

_____

_____

_____

_____

_____

_____

_____

_____

_____

_____

_____

_____

_____

_____

_____

_____

_____

_____

_____

_____

Data Sheet. Use these data to write your report on the opposite page. Use the correct headings.

Language Production and Comprehension	**(L2H)**
Speech-language sample: 120 utterances	How did you assess language production?
MLU: 3.0 words	
Analysis of conversational speech for missing grammatic features	How did you analyze the results?
Many morphologic features missing, but consider the errors of articulation	
(invent missing morphologic features, including the regular plural, possessive, prepositions)	What were the results of the analysis?
Limited sentence structures	
Tests administered: Peabody Picture Vocabulary Test	How did you assess comprehension?
The Test for Auditory Comprehension of Language (TACL)	
Language comprehension: Age appropriate (on both the tests)	What were the results?
Voice and Fluency	**(L2H)**
Informally assessed through conversational speech samples	How did you assess voice and fluency?
Judged to be within normal limits	What is your evaluation?

Write your report. Use the information on the data sheet. Invent information as needed.

_____

_____

_____

_____

_____

_____

_____

_____

_____

_____

_____

_____

_____

_____

_____

_____

_____

_____

_____

_____

_____

_____

> Data Sheet. Use these data to write your report on the opposite page. Use the correct headings.

DIAGNOSTIC SUMMARY

Multiple misarticulations

Speech intelligibility: 60%

Normal voice and fluency

Limited language structures; many missing morphologic features

RECOMMENDATIONS

Treatment recommended

Goal is to teach the misarticulated phonemes

A later, more detailed language assessment

Parent training in maintenance

Submitted by_____

Parent's signature_____

Approved by _____

(L1H)

Summarize the communicative problems.

(L1H)

Do you recommend treatment?
What are the priority treatment targets?
Who submitted the report? Write the name, degree, and title.
Parent's name and signature

Who approved the report?
Write the name, degree, certification, and title.

Write your report. Use the information on the data sheet. Invent information as needed.

_____
_____
_____
_____
_____
_____
_____
_____
_____
_____
_____
_____
_____
_____
_____
_____
_____
_____
_____
_____
_____
_____
_____
_____

C.1.5. ASSESSMENT REPORT: *LANGUAGE DISORDERS*

Data Sheet. Use these data to write your report on the opposite page. Use the correct headings.

Name of the clinic, city, and state: (invent)

(L1H)

Write the name and address of the clinic.

DIAGNOSTIC REPORT

(L1H)

What kind of report?

Sylvia Sun, client; age, 5; address: (invent); telephone: (invent); clinician: yourself; date of assessment: (invent); diagnosis: Language Disorder; referred by Dr. Chang Loongson, a physician.

Identifying information Arrange appropriately

BACKGROUND AND REASONS FOR REFERRAL

(L1H)

Date seen at the clinic (invent)
Use the information above
No prior assessment
Informant: Mrs. Katie Sun, mother

Who, how old a person, referred when, to which clinic and why?

Write your report. Use the information on the data sheet. Invent information as needed.

Data Sheet. Use these data to write your report on the opposite page. Use the correct headings.

HISTORY

Birth and Development

Normal pregnancy, delivery

No significant prenatal or natal complications

Normal infancy

Delayed language and motor development

First words at 22 months

Two-word phrases not until 28 months

Errors of articulation

"Does not speak in complete sentences" (mother)

"Does not know many words" (mother)

Medical History

One episode of high fever and convulsions at age 16 months

Prone to frequent episodes of coughs, colds, and allergic reactions

Chicken pox at 4

Slow physical growth

(L1H)

(L2H)

Prenatal, birth
Mother's health
Early development
Early language
development

(L2H)

Diseases of
significance

Write your report. Use the information on the data sheet. Invent information as needed.

Data Sheet. Use these data to write your report on the opposite page. Use the correct headings.

Family, Social, and Educational History	**(L2H)**
An older sister (8 years), a younger brother (3 years) Sister is diagnosed as developmentally delayed, enrolled in special education No parental concern about the younger brother's speech and language	Family How many children?
Older sister is language delayed, getting treated in school	Any family history of communicative problems?
Mother: a high school graduate; a receptionist in an auto body repair shop Father: high school graduate; plumber	Parent's education and occupation
Enrolled in a kindergarten program Needs special attention	Educational information
Does not play cooperatively Has a few companions who are much younger	Child's companions and social behavior
	Any other information about the family

Write your report. Use the information on the data sheet. Invent information as needed.

Data Sheet. Use these data to write your report on the opposite page. Use the correct headings.

ASSESSMENT INFORMATION	**(L1H)**
	(L2H)
Orofacial Examination	
	Describe the orofacial examination: integrity of oral and facial structures.
No malocclusion	
Sluggish lingual movements	
Slow diadochokinetic rate	Give a general description of the face, mouth, teeth, tongue, hard and soft palate, and movement of the soft palate and the tongue.
No other findings of significance	
Hearing Screening	**(L2H)**
Screened: 250, 500, 1000, 2000, 4000, and 8000 Hz at 25 dB HL	What frequencies were screened and at what level?
Passed at all tested frequencies	What were the results?

Write your report. Use the information on the data sheet. Invent information as needed.

_____

_____

_____

_____

_____

_____

_____

_____

_____

_____

_____

_____

_____

_____

_____

_____

_____

_____

_____

_____

_____

_____

_____

_____

_____

Speech Production and Intelligibility	**(L2H)**
Conversational speech sample	How was speech production assessed?
Templin-Darley Test of Articulation	
	Give the full name of tests administered. Do not ignore speech samples.
Numerous errors in both	
In the initial position of words, omitted: /b, d, t, l, g, m, n, k/; distorted: /z, s/	Summarize the errors in a table.
In the medial position of words, omitted: /b, m, f, z, s, l, g, r/	
In the final position of words, omitted: /b, d, p, r, k, t, m, n, s/	
The same errors in conversational speech	
Intelligibility with contextual cues: 80% for utterances	What was the speech intelligibility?

Write your report. Use the information on the data sheet. Invent information as needed.

Data Sheet. Use these data to write your report on the opposite page. Use the correct headings.

Language Production and Comprehension	**(L2H)**
Language sample: 60 utterances Shown pictures, objects, and toys to evoke language	How did you assess language production? What tests?
MLU: 4.0 words	
Analysis of conversational speech for missing grammatic features and pragmatic functions	How did you analyze the results?
Limited vocabulary Many morphologic features missing (invent missing morphologic features, e.g., the plural *s*, present progressive *ing*, past tense *ed*) Typically, three-to-four-word utterances Few grammatically complete sentences Limited sentence structures and few sentence varieties Difficulty in maintaining topic and in conversational turn taking	What were the results of the analysis?
The Assessment of Children's Language Comprehension (ACLC); clinical judgment during interview and language sampling Language comprehension: Approximately that of a 3-year-old	How did you assess language comprehension? What were the results?
Voice and Fluency	**(L2H)**
Informally assessed through conversational speech samples Limited fluency because of limited language Voice judged to be within normal limits	How did you assess voice and fluency? What is your evaluation?

Write your report. Use the information on the data sheet. Invent information as needed.

> Data Sheet. Use these data to write your report on the opposite page. Use the correct headings.

DIAGNOSTIC SUMMARY

(L1H)

Multiple misarticulations

Speech intelligibility: 65%

Normal voice but limited fluency

Limited vocabulary and language structures; many missing morphologic features; pragmatic problems; deficiency in language comprehension

Summarize the communicative problems.

RECOMMENDATIONS

(L1H)

Treatment recommended

Initial goal is to expand vocabulary, teach early morphemes, and basic sentence structures

Later goal is to teach correct articulation of phonemes, pragmatic features

A more detailed language assessment before initiating treatment

Parent training in a home treatment and maintenance program

Do you recommend treatment?
What are the priority treatment targets?

Submitted by_____

Who submitted the report? Write the name, degree, and title.
Parent's name and signature

Parent's signature_____
            Mrs. Katie Sun

Who approved the report?
Write the name, degree, certification, and title.

Approved by _____

Write your report. Use the information on the data sheet. Invent information as needed.

C.1.5. ASSESSMENT REPORT: *STUTTERING*

Data Sheet. Use these data to write your report on the opposite page. Use the correct headings.

Name of the clinic, city, and state: (invent)

(L1H)

Write the name and address of the clinic.

DIAGNOSTIC REPORT

(L1H)

Marvin Lenson, client; age, 32; address: (invent); telephone: (invent); clinician: yourself; date of assessment: (invent); diagnosis: stuttering; referral: self

What kind of report? Identifying information Arrange appropriately

BACKGROUND AND REASONS FOR REFERRAL

(L1H)

Use the information above

Date evaluated (invent)

Several prior assessments and treatments at various clinics with no lasting effects

Informant: Self

Client reported that: stuttering started when he was about 5 (according to his mother)

Has had prior treatment throughout the school years

Does not recall treatment techniques except that he was encouraged to think before talking

Stuttering varies across situations; but more stuttering when talking to strangers; his boss; more fluent talking to wife; avoids telephones, ordering in restaurants, and talking to groups

Who, how old a person, referred when, to which clinic and why? Summarize the history of stuttering.

Write your report. Use the information on the data sheet. Invent information as needed.

_____

_____

_____

_____

_____

_____

_____

_____

_____

_____

_____

_____

_____

_____

_____

_____

_____

_____

_____

_____

_____

_____

_____

_____

_____

_____

Data Sheet. Use these data to write your report on the opposite page. Use the correct headings.

HISTORY   (L1H)

Birth and Development   (L2H)

Mother had told the client that everything was normal   Prenatal, birth
                                                                          Mother's health
Mother's health during pregnancy reportedly normal   Early development

Normal infancy

Normal motor development

Advanced early language development as told by parents   Early language
                                                                          development
Considers himself verbally competent; likes to read and
write; has good vocabulary and command of the language

Medical History   (L2H)

Nothing of clinical significance   Diseases of
                                                                          significance

Note: In the case of most adult clients, *Birth and Development* may not
be a necessary heading. However, when there is information available or
is considered relevant for a given disorder, there is nothing wrong in
including it.

Write your report. Use the information on the data sheet. Invent information as needed.

_____

_____

_____

_____

_____

_____

_____

_____

_____

_____

_____

_____

_____

_____

_____

_____

_____

_____

_____

_____

_____

_____

_____

Data Sheet. Use these data to write your report on the opposite page. Use the correct headings.	

Family, Social, and Educational History	**(L2H)**
An older brother (37 years), a younger sister (27 years), a younger brother (24 years)	Family How many children?
Older brother used to stutter but has been mostly fluent for the past 10 years; has had unspecified treatment A maternal uncle (65) still stutters A paternal aunt (62) used to stutter but has been fluent for many years No family history of other communicative disorders	Any family history of communicative problems?
Both hold doctoral degrees Mother: a pediatrician Father: clinical psychologist	Parents' education and occupation
Client holds a master's degree in structural engineering Works for a construction company	Educational and occupational information
Married, wife owns a clothing store one daughter (3), speaks normally	Personal information

Write your report. Use the information on the data sheet. Invent information as needed.

Data Sheet. Use these data to write your report on the opposite page. Use the correct headings.

## ASSESSMENT INFORMATION	**(L1H)**
Orofacial Examination	**(L2H)**
Nothing of clinical significance	Describe the orofacial examination: integrity of oral and facial structures.
Hearing Screening	**(L2H)**
Screened: 250, 500, 1000, 2000, 4000, and 8000 Hz at 25 dB HL	What frequencies were screened and at what level?
Passed the screening	What were the results?

Write your report. Use the information on the data sheet. Invent information as needed.

Data Sheet. Use these data to write your report on the opposite page. Use the correct headings.

Speech and Language Production	**(L2H)**
Informally assessed as the client was interviewed	How were speech and language production assessed?
Judged to have normal articulation and superior language skills	
Speech intelligibility was 100% for utterances with or without knowledge of contexts	What was the speech intelligibility? Summarize the observations.
Voice	**(L2H)**
Informally assessed as the client was interviewed Vocal qualities judged to be normal	How assessed? Summarize the observations.

Write your report. Use the information on the data sheet. Invent information as needed.

_____

_____

_____

_____

_____

_____

_____

_____

_____

_____

_____

_____

_____

_____

_____

_____

_____

_____

_____

_____

_____

_____

_____

Data Sheet. Use these data to write your report on the opposite page. Use the correct headings.

Assessment of Fluency | **(L2H)**

Conversational speech sample: 2,000 words | How did you assess fluency and stuttering?

Oral reading sample: 500 words

Two home samples of at least 1,000 words each requested for later analysis

Analysis of types and frequency of dysfluencies (all types) | How did you analyze the results?

Calculation of percent dysfluency rate

Results: | What were the results of the analysis?

In conversational speech:

Part-word reps: 57; sound prolongations: 48; syllable interjections: 28; whole-word reps: 39; pauses (1 sec or more): 45; broken words: 21

Total number of dysfluencies: 238

Percent dysfluency rate: 11.9

Oral reading: | Describe the frequency and types of dysfluencies in oral reading

Part-word reps: 42; sound prolongations: 39; syllable interjections: 34; whole-word reps: 53; pauses (1 sec or more): 54; broken words: 21

Total number of dysfluencies: 243

Percent dysfluency rate: 48.6

Eye blinks, knitting of the eyebrows associated with sound prolongations and word repetitions | Describe the associated motor behaviors.

Write your report. Use the information on the data sheet. Invent information as needed.

_____

_____

_____

_____

_____

_____

_____

_____

_____

_____

_____

_____

_____

_____

_____

_____

_____

_____

_____

_____

_____

_____

_____

_____

_____

_____

_____

> Data Sheet. Use these data to write your report on the opposite page. Use the correct headings.

DIAGNOSTIC SUMMARY

(L1H)

Clinically significant dysfluency rate: 11.9%

Part-word reps, sound prolongations, syllable interjections, whole-word reps, pauses, and broken words

Higher dysfluency rate in oral reading: 48.6

Few associated motor behaviors

Summarize the dysfluency rates. Specify the types.

RECOMMENDATIONS

(L1H)

Treatment recommended

Goal is to teach the skills of fluency (gentle phonatory onset, rate reduction through syllable prolongation, and appropriate airflow management)

Self-monitoring skills for maintenance

Do you recommend treatment? What are the priority treatment targets?

Submitted by_____

Who submitted the report? Write the name, degree, and title.

Client's signature_____
            Marvin Lenson

Client's name and signature

Approved by _____

Who approved the report? Write the name, degree, certification, and title.

Write your report. Use the information on the data sheet. Invent information as needed.

C.1.5. ASSESSMENT REPORT: *VOICE DISORDER*

Data Sheet. Use these data to write your report on the opposite page. Use the correct headings.

Name of the clinic, city, and state: (invent)	**(L1H)** Write the name and address of the clinic.
DIAGNOSTIC REPORT	**(L1H)** What kind of report?
Raj Mohan, 35 years; address: (invent); telephone: (invent); clinician: yourself; date of assessment: (invent); diagnosis: Voice Disorder (Inadequate Loudness); referred by: Dr. Melanie Mallard, Otolaryngologist	Identifying information Arrange appropriately
BACKGROUND AND REASONS FOR REFERRAL	**(L1H)**
Use the information above No prior assessment; date assessed (invent) Informant: Self	Who, how old a person, referred when, to which clinic and why?
Client reports that: his voice is too soft for his occupation (high school teacher); voice gets tired too soon during the working days; students complain because of too soft voice; has had the problem for the past 2 years; not much variation	Summarize the history of the voice disorder.

Write your report. Use the information on the data sheet. Invent information as needed.

Data Sheet. Use these data to write your report on the opposite page. Use the correct headings.

HISTORY

(L1H)

Birth and Development

(L2H)

No relevant information; eliminate this heading in the report

Medical History

(L2H)

ENT report negative; normal laryngeal structures

No medical basis for the symptoms

ENT recommends voice treatment

Diseases of significance

Write your report. Use the information on the data sheet. Invent information as needed.

Data Sheet. Use these data to write your report on the opposite page. Use the correct headings.

Family, Social, and Educational History	**(L2H)**
.	
The only child in the family	Family How many children?
No history of voice disorder or other communicative disorders	Any family history of communicative problems?
Mother: college graduate; a college counselor Father: college graduate; a college admissions officer	Parents' education and occupation

Write your report. Use the information on the data sheet. Invent information as needed.

Data Sheet. Use these data to write your report on the opposite page. Use the correct headings.

ASSESSMENT INFORMATION

(L1H)

Orofacial Examination

(L2H)

Negative (means nothing of clinical significance)

Describe the orofacial examination: integrity of oral and facial structures.

Hearing Screening

(L2H)

Screened: 250, 500, 1000, 2000, 4000, and 8000 Hz at 25 dB HL

What frequencies were screened and at what level?

Passed at all frequencies

What were the results?

Write your report. Use the information on the data sheet. Invent information as needed.

| Data Sheet. Use these data to write your report on the opposite page. Use the correct headings. |

Speech, Language, and Fluency

Based on the observation of conversational speech during interview, judged to be within normal limits

Speech 100% intelligible with or without contextual knowledge

(L2H)

How were they assessed?

What was the speech intelligibility?

Write your report. Use the information on the data sheet. Invent information as needed.

Data Sheet. Use these data to write your report on the opposite page. Use the correct headings.

Voice

	(L2H)
Subjectively rated on a 5–point scale from very soft to very loud (1 = very soft; 5 = very loud)	How was voice assessed?
Received a rating of 2, soft voice	
Also measured with a sound level meter with the microphone placed at 8 inches from the client's face	What were the results?
Measurement showed 45 dB, judged too soft	
Additional data: in each class period, the client's students request some five to six times to speak louder	
Was asked to baserate the frequency with which the students request him to speak louder over 5 consecutive days	

Write your report. Use the information on the data sheet. Invent information as needed.

_____

_____

_____

_____

_____

_____

_____

_____

_____

_____

_____

_____

_____

_____

_____

_____

_____

_____

_____

_____

_____

_____

_____

_____

_____

> Data Sheet. Use these data to write your report on the opposite page. Use the correct headings.

DIAGNOSTIC SUMMARY   **(L1H)**

Self-report, clinical judgment, and instrumental measurement suggest a voice that is too soft to meet the demands of the client's social and occupational life

Summarize the voice disorder.

RECOMMENDATIONS   **(L1H)**

Treatment recommended

Shape a louder voice considered appropriate for classroom teaching

Reduce or eliminate the number of student requests to speak louder by shaping appropriately louder voice

Do you recommend treatment?
What are the priority treatment targets?

Submitted by_____

Who submitted the report?
Write the name, degree, and title.

Client's signature_____
       Raj Mohan

Client's name and signature

Approved by _____

Who approved the report?
Write the name, degree, certification, and title.

Write your report. Use the information on the data sheet. Invent information as needed.

_____

_____

_____

_____

_____

_____

_____

_____

_____

_____

_____

_____

_____

_____

_____

_____

_____

_____

_____

_____

_____

_____

_____

Note to Student Clinician

Contact your clinic secretary for additional examples of assessment reports. Take note of variations in formats. Practice writing reports according to your clinic format. Use the practice formats presented in this section.

C.1.6. REPORTS WRITTEN AS LETTERS TO A REFERRING PROFESSIONAL

In many clinical settings, especially in private speech and hearing clinics, a diagnostic report may be written as a letter to a referring professional. For instance, a physician might refer a man with laryngectomy to a speech-language pathologist who then writes a letter to the physician and summarizes the assessment information.

Another reason to write an assessment report in the form of a letter is to make a referral to a specialist whose recommendation is needed before treatment may be started. For instance, a woman with a hoarse voice might consult a speech-language pathologist. The clinician that evaluates her should refer this client to a laryngologist for a laryngeal examination. In this letter, the clinician may summarize the results of voice evaluation. Treatment is begun only after the laryngeal examination does not contraindicate voice therapy.

Assessment reports written in the form of a letter to a referring professional contain only the most important facts. It is assumed that the professional who has referred the client to you has on file the details about the patient. Another professional who receives a referral is expected to obtain necessary information from the client. Therefore, the speech-language clinician need not write about the client's personal, family, and medical history. Instead, the clinician will limit the report to the most essential elements of his or her assessment and recommendations. In some cases, however, the letter that makes a referral to another professional also is the only assessment report kept in the speech and hearing clinic's file. Such letters may contain additional information about the client and his or her history of the communicative problem. Two examples follow.

Sierra Speech and Hearing Center
Johnsonville, Wyoming

SPEECH-LANGUAGE EVALUATION

April xx, xxxx

June Johnson, M.D.
Johnson Medical Group
Johnsonville, WY

RE: Victor Valence

Dear Dr. Johnson:

Thank you for referring Mr. Victor Valence, a 72-year-old male, for a speech-language assessment. I saw Mr. Valence at our clinic for a speech evaluation and consultation on April xx, xxxx. I understand that Mr. Valence was diagnosed with throat cancer approximately 3 years ago. At that time, he received radiation therapy. Because this treatment was not successful in controlling his cancer, Mr. Valence underwent a total laryngectomy on December xx, xxxx.

His wife accompanied him to the session. Mr. and Mrs. Valence both have significant hearing losses. Mr. Valence owns a hearing aid, which he does not wear. Since his laryngectomy, Mr. Valence has been communicating with writing and gesture. No feeding or swallowing problems were reported.

Oral-Peripheral Examination

An oral-peripheral examination revealed adequate functioning for the production of speech sounds. Diadochokinetic rates were within normal limits. Mr. Valence's cannula had been removed and his stoma appeared to be healing well.

Electronic Speech Devices

Several electronic speech devices were available for Mr. Valence to see and try. These devices included: the Cooper Rand Intra-Oral Electrolarynx, the Romet Electrolarynx, the Western Electric Electrolarynx, the Aurex/Neovox Electrolarynx, and the Servox Electrolarynx (neck devices). Mr. Valence was no longer experiencing tenderness and pain in the neck area, so a neck device was utilized. Instructions were provided on the placement of the Aurex and on compensatory articulation strategies needed to use it. Mr. Valence was then given this electronic larynx to use at home until one of his own could be purchased. He was told to place the electrolarynx on his cheek if he experienced any neck pain or tenderness. In addition, forms were completed to obtain a free electrolarynx from the Phone Company to be used as a back-up device in the future.

Esophageal Speech

The altered anatomy and physiology of the pharynx, trachea, and esophagus and their relationship to the production of speech sounds were discussed and visually demonstrated for Mr. Valence. Esophageal speech sound production was then attempted using the following air intake methods: injection, inhalation, and plosive injection. Mr. Valence was successful in producing sound via the consonant injection and plosive injection methods. He could produce a variety of syllables and words.

Tracheo-Esophageal Puncture

Because you had suggested the possibility of a tracheo-esophageal (TE) puncture to Mr. Valence, I discussed this procedure in detail. Using pictures and drawings, I explained the surgical procedure. I showed Mr. Valence samples of various prostheses and discussed with him procedures for care and management of the TE puncture and prosthesis. Mr. and Mrs. Valence were both enthusiastic about this speech option. In my opinion, Mr. Valence's relatively good health, dexterity, motivation, independence in caring for his stoma, ability to produce esophageal phonation, and favorable disposition toward this procedure make him an excellent candidate. In addition, the size, location, and shape of his stoma are consistent with successful placement of a TE puncture.

Additional Information

I gave Mr. Valence information on ordering such supplies as stoma covers, filters, dickies, and mock turtleneck shirts. I also told him about the "Lost Chord Club" and the support he and his wife might receive from the organization.

Summary and Recommendation

Mr. Valence was highly motivated to develop a form of verbal communication, primarily with a TE puncture. He also is interested in using an electrolarynx. He demonstrated excellent potential for the use of a TE puncture and good beginning skills for the use of an electronic larynx. Therefore, I recommend that Mr. Valence receive speech treatment for a minimum of two times a week for an initial period of 3 months. The treatment will emphasize functional communication with a voice prosthesis (if the TE puncture procedure is done) and an electrolarynx. If a TE puncture is not done, the development of esophageal speech will be pursued.

Thank you for referring this patient to our center. Please contact me if you have questions or comments.

Yours sincerely,

Francine Maxtor, M.A., CCC-SLP
Speech-Language Pathologist

Northeast Speech and Hearing Center
Albany, New York

March xx, xxxx

Bart Barkley, M.D.
Albany Medical Associates

RE: Mrs. Zenner Zantosh

Dear Dr. Barkley:

I am referring Mrs. Zantosh, a 58-year-old female, to you for a medical examination. I saw Mrs. Zantosh on March x, xxxx for an assessment of her voice. The presenting complaints were hoarseness and weakness of the voice, especially when singing. The onset of her dysphonia was approximately 2 years ago. Her voice production, however, deteriorated in January, xxxx. An indirect laryngoscopy done on February xx, xxxx was negative. Mrs. Zantosh, who has recently moved to Albany, has sought treatment for her persistent dysphonia.

History[1]

Mrs. Zantosh reports a history of chronic laryngitis secondary to smoking. Eighteen years ago, Mrs. Zantosh was diagnosed as having leukoplakia and quit smoking at that time. History is negative for alcoholic beverage consumption. Mrs. Zantosh reportedly drinks two to three cups of coffee daily, eats spicy foods, uses salt frequently, and eats dairy products occasionally. Mrs. Zantosh said that she drinks approximately two to three glasses of water each day.

Mrs. Zantosh takes Seldane BID for her allergies and periodically has post-nasal drainage. Additional prescription drugs, which have been prescribed, include Synthroid and Naprosin. She reports hypothyroidism and tonsillectomy in childhood. Mrs. Zantosh states that her most recent case of laryngitis was in May 1995. Previous audiometric testing indicated a mild to moderate hearing loss in her left ear, which was identified approximately 3 years ago.

Mrs. Zantosh is employed as a teacher at McLane High School and has taught chorus at the school. Her history is positive for talking in noise at work and in the car, yelling and cheering, loud laughter, and loud and excessive talking over long periods. Telephone usage is reportedly minimal. However, until recently, Mrs. Zantosh sang in choir at church and was involved in group singing performances. Mrs. Zantosh says that she is typically hoarse following singing and has a weak voice when she is trying to sing at the middle and lower registers. She reported that her frustration with her reduced ability to sing has caused her stress.

Because she lives alone, Mrs. Zantosh experiences routine periods of vocal rest. She occasionally uses throat lozenges to alleviate the sensation of a dry throat from singing.

---

[1]Because Dr. Barkley has not seen Mrs. Zantosh before, he has no file on her and thus needs a brief case history.

Assessment Information

Mrs. Zantosh was responsive and cooperative throughout the evaluation period. The results appeared to be indicative of her typical vocal behavior.

Vocally Abusive Behaviors: During the assessment session, Mrs. Zantosh cleared her throat 16 times. She also exhibited several instances of hard glottal attacks.

Vocal Parameters: Vocal quality was noted to be intermittently harsh, with a low vocal pitch. An elevated loudness level also was evident. Nonetheless, during assessment, her overall pitch and loudness ranges appeared to be within normal limits. Mrs. Zantosh occasionally produced pitch breaks and exhibited vocal fry at the ends of her sentences. A deterioration in her voice was noted across an oral reading passage. She was able to prolong the /s/ sound for 31 seconds and prolonged /z/ for 38 seconds. Both of these results were within normal limits.

Physical Parameters: Mrs. Zantosh maintained a forward head position during the evaluation. Additionally, she complained of tension in her shoulders. Oral mobility was good.

Trial Therapy: Mrs. Zantosh could produce a clear voice following the clinician's instructions to raise her pitch. With modeling, she also could exhibit gentle phonatory onset.

Oral-Peripheral Exam: An inspection of the patient's oral-facial complex revealed structures and functions to be within normal limits.

Summary and Recommendations

Mrs. Zantosh presents a clinically significant voice disorder, characterized by a harsh quality, low pitch, and reportedly increased vocal loudness. Additionally, she engages in several vocally abusive behaviors. It is recommended that she receive intensive voice therapy on a twice-a-week basis for approximately 3 months. Her prognosis for improvement is good. Because her role as a teacher places such demands on voice production, it is vital that she receive voice therapy immediately to improve her voice and to prevent any further deterioration in her vocal skills.

The following treatment objectives are appropriate:

1. Train Mrs. Zantosh to produce a clear vocal quality at a conversational level across persons, settings, and situations.

2. Increase vocal pitch.

3. Reduce loudness during conversation.

4. Eliminate pitch breaks and vocal fry.

5. Improve head positioning during speech.

I am referring Mrs. Zantosh to you for a medical examination prior to initiating voice treatment. If you have questions or suggestions about the proposed plan of treatment, please contact me. I look forward to receiving a copy of your report.

Yours sincerely,

Janet Jackson, Ph.D., CCC-SLP
Speech-Language Pathologist

Note to Student Clinicians

Reports written as letters vary greatly in details and the use of jargon, depending on the recipient. The examples given are only samples. Therefore, find out the format and content of letters your clinic may send to insurance companies, government agencies, and private organizations that fund speech, language, and hearing services. Some of these offices may receive printed forms that the clinic fills out and sends for reimbursement.

C.I.7. PRACTICE IN WRITING REPORTS AS LETTERS

C.1.7. ASSESSMENT REPORT AS A LETTER: *ARTICULATION DISORDER*

On the next page, write a letter to a referring pediatrician summarizing your assessment of a child with an articulation disorder. The pediatrician referred the child to you, and you are reporting your assessment results.

Data Sheet. Use these data to write your report on the opposite page. Use the correct headings.

Your Clinic's name and address (invent)	**(L1H)** Use the standard letter format
Date The pediatrician's name and address (invent) RE: The child's name (invent) Salutation:	
Use the following information to construct a letter No need to use headings or subheadings Child, 8 years old Mother brought the child to the clinic No significant medical, prenatal, natal, or developmental history Has an older brother and a younger sister (invent their ages) No family history of communicative disorders Doing well in school	Brief history
Orofacial examination revealed structure and function within normal limits	Orofacial examination

Write your report. Use the information on the data sheet. Invent information as needed.

_____

_____

_____

_____

_____

_____

_____

_____

_____

_____

_____

_____

_____

_____

_____

_____

_____

_____

_____

_____

_____

_____

_____

_____

Data Sheet. Use these data to write your report on the opposite page. Use the correct headings.	

Goldman-Fristoe Test of Articulation Conversational speech sample Various errors of articulation including omissions and substitutions (invent)	Assessment methods and results
No language, voice, or fluency problems (informally assessed during the interview)	Comments on other aspects of communication
Treatment is recommended Suggest the treatment goals	Treatment information
Thank you, call me and so forth	Concluding remarks
Type your name Sign your name	Your name, degree, and signature

Write your report. Use the information on the data sheet. Invent information as needed.

Note to Student Clinicians

Think of other kinds of letters clinicians might write. Contact your clinic director to find out what kinds of letters are routinely sent out by the clinic.

C.2. TREATMENT PLANS

The treatment plans written for clients vary across professional settings. The plans written in university clinics are perhaps more detailed than those that are written at other settings. A student who learns to write detailed and comprehensive treatment plans can easily write less extensive and briefer reports. Examples of more and less detailed treatment plans follow.

Treatment plans, like assessment reports, need not follow the APA format in every respect. Heading styles will vary; the examples that follow use different styles to illustrate this variety. One-sentence paragraphs, lists (incomplete sentences), and other deviations from the APA style may be acceptable in treatment plans, especially in those that are brief.

Student clinicians are encouraged to see these varied forms and styles as intended reflection of practice across clinics. The variations should not be thought of as inconsistencies. Student clinicians need to find out the accepted format in their clinic by talking to their clinic director and clinical supervisor.

C.2.1. COMPREHENSIVE TREATMENT PLANS

Some supervisors may ask you to write a comprehensive treatment plan for your client. A comprehensive treatment plan is more detailed than a brief treatment plan, which often is described as a lesson plan. Such a detailed treatment plan includes the following components:

1. A brief summary of previous assessment data
2. Treatment targets
3. Treatment and probe procedures
4. Maintenance program
5. Follow-up and booster treatment procedures

A student who writes a comprehensive treatment plan understands the total management program for a client. The student may or may not complete the program in a semester or quarter. Nonetheless, writing a comprehensive treatment program is a good exercise in visualizing the entire treatment sequence from the beginning to the end. Beyond clinical practicum, this is what clinicians do in professional setting. After assessing their clients, clinicians develop comprehensive treatment plans for them. Therefore, although the student clinicians complete only a portion of a treatment plan, it is desirable to think of the total treatment program for a client.

C.2.1. COMPREHENSIVE TREATMENT PLAN: *ARTICULATION DISORDER*

University Speech and Hearing Clinic

TREATMENT PLAN

Name: Oliver Driver
Date of Birth: xx-xx-xxxx
Address: 312 N. South #111
City: Martinsville, CA 64812
School: University Preschool

Diagnosis: Articulation Disorder
File no.: 900111-3
Semesters in Therapy: 1
Date of Report: xx-xx-xxxx
Telephone: 782-9832

BACKGROUND INFORMATION

Oliver Driver, a 4-year-old male, began his first semester of speech treatment at the University Speech and Hearing Clinic in February, xxxx. Oliver's speech and language were evaluated on January 15, xxxx. The evaluation revealed an articulation disorder characterized by substitutions, omissions, and reduced intelligibility. See his folder for a diagnostic report. Treatment was recommended to train correct production of misarticulated phonemes to increase speech intelligibility. Based on Oliver's cooperative behavior during assessment, prognosis for improved articulation was judged good.

TARGET BEHAVIORS

The **final target** for Oliver is to produce all phonemes correctly in conversational speech with at least 90% accuracy.

The **initial target** is to produce selected phonemes correctly. Based on their inconsistent production during assessment, the following phonemes were selected for the initial treatment: /p/, /m/, /s/, /k/, and /g/. Production of each phoneme was baserated with 20 stimulus words administered on modeled and evoked discrete trials with the following correct baseline response rates:

Phonemes	Evoked	Modeled
/p/:	15%	17%
/m/:	10%	24%
/s/:	12%	22%
/k/:	18%	20%
/g/:	14%	17%

Treatment was begun after obtaining the baserates. The following general treatment procedures will be used during the semester. The procedures will be modified as suggested by Oliver's performance data. These changes will be described in the final progress report.

TREATMENT AND PROBE PROCEDURES

Each target phoneme will initially be trained at the word level. When Oliver's probe response rate at the word level meets a 90% correct criterion, training will be initiated on two-word phrases. A similar probe criterion will be used to shift training to sentences and then to conversational speech.

Intermixed probes on which trained and untrained words, phrases, or sentences are alternated will be administered every time Oliver meets a tentative training criterion of 90% correct response rate on a block of 20 evoked training trials. Oliver will be trained to meet this criterion at each level of response topography (words, phrases, and sentences).

Initially, the clinician will provide stimulus pictures. Subsequently, Oliver will be required to find at least five pictures in magazines that represent the target sound and bring them to the clinic sessions. After he correctly produces a target sound on five consecutive trials, he will paste a picture that represents the just trained sound in a book. This book will be used for both clinic and home practice.

Training will begin at each level with discrete trials and modeling. The clinician will show Oliver a picture, ask a question ("What is this?") and model the response (word or phrase). Oliver will then be required to imitate the clinician's production. When Oliver correctly imitates the target sound on five consecutive trials, modeling will be discontinued. The clinician will show Oliver a picture and ask, "What is this?" to evoke a response.

At the modeled and evoked word levels, verbal reinforcement will be administered on an FR1 schedule for correct productions. At the phrase and sentence levels, an FR4 will be used. At the conversational level, verbal reinforcement will be delivered on an approximate VR5 schedule. All incorrect productions at each level will immediately be interrupted by saying, "stop."

Modeling will be reintroduced if Oliver gives two to four incorrect responses on the evoked trials. Shaping with manual guidance will be used as necessary.
The clinician will chart all productions in all treatment sessions. Oliver also will chart productions with an X under the *happy face* (correct responses) or X under the *sad face* (incorrect responses). At the end of each session, Oliver will assist the clinician in recording his progress on a graph.

It is expected that different target sounds will reach the training criterion at different times. Therefore, the clinician expects to train several sounds at different response topographies in each session. Some sounds may be trained at the word level while others may be trained at the phrase or even sentence level. When the initially selected target sounds meet the criterion of 90% correct probe rate in conversational speech in the clinic, new target sounds will be baserated and trained.

MAINTENANCE PROGRAM

After Oliver produces the target sound with 90% accuracy at the evoked word level, his mother, Mrs. Janice Driver, will be asked to participate in treatment. Initially, she will observe the treatment procedure. Soon, Mrs. Driver will be trained to present stimulus items and chart correct and incorrect productions. She will be trained to immediately reinforce the correct productions and stopping Oliver at the earliest sign of an inaccurate production.

After Oliver's mother identifies correct and incorrect responses with at least 80% accuracy in the clinic session, she will be trained to work with him at home. Mrs. Driver will begin with such structured activities as reciting from a list or reading from the book he will be developing in treatment. Assignments will progress to monitoring and recording speech during dinner and phone conversations with Oliver's grandmother, who will be encouraged to prompt and then praise the correct productions. The clinician, Oliver, and his mother will review tape-recorded home assignments. The mother will be given feedback on the procedures implemented at home.

When Oliver produces the target sound with 90% accuracy in conversation in the sessions, he will be taken out of the clinic to practice correct productions in nonclinical situations. The clinician will take Oliver for a walk on campus and talk with him. Subsequently, he may be taken to the campus bookstore, library, cafeteria, and other places. Eventually, his speech may be monitored informally in shopping centers and restaurants.

When Oliver's speech is 98% intelligible and his sound productions are 90% correct, he may be dismissed from treatment. A follow-up visit will be scheduled for 6 months after dismissal. Based on the initial follow-up results, booster treatment, treatment for persistent errors, or additional follow-up assessments will be planned.

Submitted by: _____
        Marla Model, B.A.
        Student Clinician

Parent's signature: _____

Approved by: _____
        Barbara Sierra, M.S., CCC/SP
        Clinical Supervisor

C.2.2. BRIEF TREATMENT PLANS

Brief or short-term treatment plans, also known as lesson plans, are probably used more frequently. The scope of these plans varies across clinics and supervisors. Some plans describe what will be done in only a session or two. Others might describe treatment objectives and procedures planned for a week, a quarter, or a semester. Even those plans that describe the plan for a semester may not be as comprehensive as a complete treatment plan. In some plans, only the treatment objectives may be listed. However, all treatment plans—long or short—should contain a statement of prognosis and a description of target behaviors, treatment procedures, and performance criteria.

The examples of brief treatment plans given on the following pages show slightly different formats in which they may be written. The sampling of formats is not comprehensive; the examples suggest a few basic variations. Heading styles and paragraph formats are varied purposefully.

C.2.2. BRIEF TREATMENT PLAN: *FLUENCY DISORDER*

Speech and Hearing Clinic
Eastern State University
Bedford, California

James Foxx, a 23-year-old male, was seen on February x, xxxx, for a speech evaluation at the Speech and Hearing Clinic of Eastern State University, Bedford, California. The results of the evaluation indicated a severe fluency disorder with 21% dysfluency rate in conversational speech. His dysfluencies are characterized by repetitions, prolongations, pauses, interjections, and revisions. A fluency treatment program was recommended. With consistent treatment, prognosis for improved fluency was judged good.

A fluency-shaping program was selected for James. The program consists of the following final treatment objective and specific target fluency skills:

Final Treatment Objective: A dysfluency rate that does not exceed 5% in James's home and other nonclinical settings.

TARGET BEHAVIORS

1. **Appropriate management of airflow.** To produce and sustain fluency in conversational speech, James will be taught to inhale and then immediately exhale a slight amount of air before phonation. He also will be taught to sustain smooth flow of air throughout his utterances.
2. **Gentle onset of phonation.** James will be taught to initiate phonation in a soft and easy manner.
3. **Reduced speech rate through syllable prolongation.** James will be taught to prolong vowels to reduce his speech rate and to achieve continuous phonation.
4. **Continuous phonation.** Throughout an utterance, James will be taught to maintain continuous phonation by not pausing between words.
5. **Normal prosody.** Maintenance of normal prosodic features with a dysfluency rate that does not exceed 5%.

TREATMENT PROCEDURES

1. A baseline of dysfluency rates and speech rate in conversational speech will be established before starting the treatment.
2. Treatment will begin at the phrase or short sentence level.
3. The target fluency skills will be taught one at a time, beginning with inhalation and slight exhalation. Gentle onset will then be added, followed by syllable prolongation and other target skills.
4. As James sustains 98% stutter-free speech at each level of response complexity, utterance length will be increased.

5. The clinician will give instructions and model target responses consistently in the beginning stages and as often as necessary in subsequent stages of treatment.
6. The clinician will verbally reinforce the production of all target behaviors including the resulting fluency.
7. The clinician will give corrective feedback for incorrect responses, including dysfluencies; this feedback will be given at the earliest sign of a dysfluency or mismanagement of a target fluency skill.
8. When James sustains speech with 2% or less dysfluency, normal prosodic features will be trained by having him increase his speech rate and by using normal intonational patterns.
9. As James sustains 98% fluency in conversational speech, maintenance procedures will be implemented. James's wife and a colleague of his will be trained in evoking and reinforcing skills of fluency. James will be taught to self-monitor his fluency skills. The clinician will take James to extraclinical situations to evoke and reinforce his fluency skills. Home speech samples will be used to judge maintenance of fluency.
10. Follow-up will be scheduled for 3, 6, and 12 months postdismissal. Booster treatment will be arranged as needed.

Signature:_____
        Gloria Marquez, B.A.
        Student Clinician

        I understand the results of the evaluation and agree to the recommended treatment plan.

Signature:_____   Date:_____
        James Foxx

Signature:_____
        Henriette Bordern Ph.D., CCC-SLP
        Speech-Language Pathologist, Supervisor

C.2.2. BRIEF TREATMENT PLAN: *ARTICULATION DISORDER*

Valley Speech and Hearing Center
Nordstrom, Maine

Rudy Amos, a 7-year-old boy, was referred to the Valley Speech and Hearing Center for assessment and treatment of an articulation disorder. According to an assessment made on February xx, xxxx, Rudy has an articulation disorder limited to omissions of the following phonemes in both the word initial and final positions: /k, l, s, t, r/, and /z/. Treatment was recommended. Prognosis for improvement was judged excellent because Rudy was readily stimulable and highly cooperative during a brief period of trial therapy.

The treatment was begun on February xx, xxxx. A baserate showed 0 to 10% accuracy on the target phonemes. The baserates on modeled and evoked trials were similar.

The treatment will have the following final goal, specific objectives, and procedures.

Final treatment goal: Correct production of target phonemes maintained in conversational speech produced in the natural environment with at least a 90% accuracy.

Objective 1. Correct production of misarticulated phonemes in the initial, medial, and final word positions with a minimum of 90% accuracy.

Procedures: Pictures that help evoke words with the target sounds in the three positions will be used. Instructions, demonstrations, and visual feedback will be used as found necessary. If necessary, various sound-shaping techniques will be used. All correct responses will be modeled. A shaping procedure will be used to refine the production of each target phoneme. Rudy will be verbally reinforced for all imitated responses. Corrective feedback will be given for incorrect responses.

When Rudy meets the training criterion of 90% correct on words, an intermixed probe will be conducted. The probe criterion will be 90% correct production of each target phoneme in 20 untrained words. Training and probe will be alternated until this criterion is met.

Objective 2. Correct production of misarticulated phonemes in phrases and sentences.

Procedures: Training will be shifted to phrase level when Rudy meets the probe criterion for words and to the sentence level when his responses with phrases meet the probe criterion. Picture description and controlled conversation will be used to evoke target phrases and sentences. Modeling will be provided as needed. Correct responses will be reinforced on a variable schedule designed to progressively reduce the amount of feedback. Corrective feedback will be given for all incorrect responses.

Objective 3. Correct production of misarticulated phonemes in conversational speech with varied audience.

Procedures: Initially, the clinician will evoke conversational speech and model and reinforce correct productions. When Rudy's accuracy of production in conversational speech reaches at least 80%, other persons will serve as the audience.

Objective 4. Correct production of target phonemes in extraclinical situations.

Procedures: Rudy will be taken out of the treatment room to various settings on the campus to strengthen the correct production of the target phonemes. Correct productions will be prompted and reinforced in a subtle manner in such places as the campus bookstore and restaurants.

Objective 5. Training Rudy's mother to evoke and reinforce correct productions in conversational speech at home.

Procedures: The mother will be asked to initially observe the sessions and later participate in the treatment sessions. She will be trained in recognizing the correct productions and in immediately praising Rudy. She will be asked to hold brief and informal treatment sessions at home. Taped home-speech samples will be used to assess the correct production of phonemes at home.

The dismissal criterion: A 90% or better correct production of the target phonemes in conversational speech produced in extraclinical situations. Periodic home-speech samples, recorded by the mother, will be used to assess this criterion.

The procedure will be modified as found necessary during the treatment sessions.

Follow-up evaluations will be conducted 3, 6, and 12 months after the dismissal. Booster treatment will be scheduled as needed.

Signed:_____
         Mohamed Ali, M.A., CCC-SLP
         Speech-Language Pathologist

I understand the treatment program, and I agree to it.

Signed:_____   Date:_____
         Mrs. Lydia Amos
         Mother

C.2.2. BRIEF TREATMENT PLAN: *LANGUAGE DISORDER*

Speech and Hearing Clinic
Southern State University
Johnstonville, Louisiana

Timothy Krebs, a 4-year-old boy, was evaluated at the Speech and Hearing Clinic at the Southern State University on February x, xxxx. The evaluation revealed a severe language disorder. Case history and assessment data showed that his language performance is limited to a few words and phrases. A detailed assessment report can be found in Timothy's file. A language treatment program was recommended.

Timothy will be seen two times weekly in sessions lasting 45 min. His mother, Mrs. Anne Krebs, will accompany him to the clinic and will participate in treatment sessions. It is judged that prognosis for improved language performance is good if the treatment is consistent and that a home treatment and maintenance program is sustained. The following treatment objectives were selected for this semester (Fall, xxxx).

INITIAL TREATMENT OBJECTIVES

Correct production of selected functional words at 90% accuracy.

With the help of Timothy's mother, the following 20 targets consisting of single words or two-word phrases of high functional value were selected for initial treatment:

cup	sock	milk	shoe	Jenny (sister)
juice	more	eat	give me	walking
no more	I want	cookie	candy	bath
shirt	look!	Hi	Binny (dog)	John (friend)

Timothy did not produce any of these words on evoked or modeled baseline trials.

SUBSEQUENT TREATMENT OBJECTIVES

Correct Production of Additional Words

Expansion of Single Words into Phrases and Sentences

Production of Early Morphological Features (present progressive, regular plural, possessive, prepositions, pronouns, etc.)

INITIAL TREATMENT PROCEDURES

1. Pictures, objects, toys, acted-out situations, and role-playing will be used as stimuli to evoke the target words or phrases.
2. The clinician and the mother will take turns in evoking the target words or phrases.
3. Initially, gross approximations will be reinforced by verbal praise and such natural reinforcers as handing an object, complying with a request, and so forth. Subsequently, only better approximations will be reinforced.
4. All correct and incorrect productions will be measured in each treatment session.
5. When single words meet the training criterion of 90% accuracy across two sessions, intermixed probes will be expanded into phrases and then to simple sentences.
6. The mother will be asked to conduct similar treatment sessions at home and bring taped samples of sessions for evaluation and feedback.

SUBSEQUENT TREATMENT PROCEDURES

1. Additional words, selected in consultation with the mother, will be trained using the same procedure described under initial treatment procedures.
2. Additional words will be expanded into phrases and sentences.
3. Selected morphologic features will be initially trained in words and later expanded into phrases and sentences.

It is expected that Timothy will need extended treatment and that both the treatment objectives and procedures will be modified in light of his performance data. The mother's participation in training from the beginning will help maintenance. A more complete maintenance program will be developed later.

Signed:_____

     Trisha Muniz, B.A.
     Student Clinician

I understand the results of the evaluation and agree to the recommended treatment plan.

Signed:_____

     Mrs. Anne Krebs

Signed:_____ Date:_____

     Maya Real, M.A., CCC-SLP
     Speech-Language Pathologist and Clinical Supervisor

C.2.2. BRIEF TREATMENT PLAN: *VOICE DISORDER*

The Sunshine speech and Hearing Center
Zingsville, Vermont

Roshana Hersh, a 21-year-old female college student, was seen at the Sunshine Speech and Hearing Center on March xx, xxxx for a voice evaluation. The evaluation suggested a pattern of vocal abuse associated with a persistent hoarseness of voice, low pitch, and socially inappropriate intensity. Her vocal abuse consists mainly of excessive talking over the telephone and shouting at children she supervises as a teacher's aid in a kindergarten school. The detailed case history and assessment data can be found in her file. A treatment program to improve her voice quality was recommended. Considering her high degree of motivation for improvement that she expressed during the interview, prognosis was judged good.

TREATMENT TARGETS

Goal 1: Production of clear voice at least 90% of the time Roshana speaks by reducing the hoarseness of voice
Objective 1a. Reduced amount of talking over the phone
Objective 1b. Reduced amount of shouting at the school

Goal 2: Increased vocal pitch
Objective 2a. Higher pitch at the level of words and phrases
Objective 2b. Higher pitch at the level of conversational speech

Goal 3: Decreased vocal intensity
Objective 3a. Softer voice at the level of words and phrases
Objective 3b. Softer voice at the level of conversational speech

TREATMENT PROCEDURES

Objectives 1a and 1b. During the first week, the frequency and durations of Roshana's telephone conversation will be baserated. She will be asked to keep a diary to record the number of daily telephone conversations and their durations. During the second week, Roshana will be asked to reduce by 10% the amount of telephone conversation time. She may achieve this by either reducing the frequency of telephone conversations or only their durations. She will continue to record the frequency and duration of telephone conversations. In subsequent weeks, she will be asked to progressively decrease the amount of time spent on telephone until the duration is reduced by about 50%.

The frequency of shouting also will be similarly baserated. Roshana will then be asked to reduce the frequency of shouting behavior in 10% decrements until the frequency approaches zero.

Objectives 2a and 2b. The Visi-Pitch will be used to shape a higher pitch consistent with Roshana's gender and age. The treatment will start at the word and phrase level and move on to conversational speech level.

Objectives 3a and 3b. The Visi-Pitch will be used to progressively decrease the vocal intensity until it is clinically judged to be appropriate for Roshana. The treatment will start at the word and phrase level and move to conversational speech level.

A maintenance program which includes an analysis of speech samples from home and periodic follow-up and booster treatment will be implemented.

Signed:_____
　　　　　Pero Boss, B.A.
　　　　　Student Clinician

I understand the results of the evaluation and agree to the recommended treatment plan.

Client's Signature:_____
　　　　　Roshana Hersh

Signed:_____
　　　　　Moss Nero, M.A., CCC-SLP
　　　　　Speech-Language Pathologist and Clinical Supervisor

Date:_____

C.2.3. INDIVIDUALIZED EDUCATIONAL PROGRAMS

In public schools, clinicians are required by law to develop individualized educational programs or family service plans. Clinicians in a typical university or hospital speech and hearing clinic essentially do the same. Individual treatment plans described so far are comparable to individualized educational programs.

Clinicians often do not have time to write lengthy or narrative treatment plans for the children they serve. Therefore, most public school clinicians use printed forms to select treatment targets for the children they treat. Formats vary across school districts, some being more detailed than others. In this section, a few examples of printed individualized education plans for speech-language services are provided.

Central Coast Unified School District
Individualized Educational Plan for Speech and Language Services

ORAL LANGUAGE AND VERBAL EXPRESSION

Student's Name_____ Birthdate_____

School _____ Grade _____ Date_____

Speech-Language Pathologist _____

Criteria for Placement: _____

Goal: To improve oral language and verbal expression.

Present Level of Performance: *See assessment report*	Target Date	Met On (Date)	Not Met
Objectives: By _6/96_ the student will complete the following objectives with 90% accuracy as measured by pre- and posttests, specialist's observations, client-specific procedures, or other procedures (specify): _____ _____ _____ _____			
Improve Oral Language through:			
Social Interaction with others: (Check the targets selected)			
1. ✓ verbally respond when spoken to	12/95		
2. ✓ verbally express feelings and needs	2/96		
3. ___ give personal information upon request			
4. ✓ ask and answer questions	4/96		
5. ___ initiate conversation			
6. ___ share personal experiences			
7. ✓ describe events in detail	5/96		
8. ___ report factual information			
9. ___ interact verbally with others			
10. ___ give sequential, accurate verbal directions			
11. ✓ take part in class discussions and reports	6/96		
12. ___ other _____			

Atlantic Unified School District
Language, Speech, and Hearing
Individualized Educational Program Objectives

TREATMENT OF ARTICULATION

Pupil _____   Speech-Language and Hearing Specialist

Date _____

School _____   Services started on _____

_____

Goal: Improved intelligibility of speech through correct production of phonemes at 90% accuracy.

Target Date	Objectives (Check the ones selected)	Evaluation and Treatment Procedures	Date Objectives Met
	Articulation		
	Correct production of the following phonemes:	Paired stimuli method of treatment	
	/d/, /t/, /p/, /ʒ/, and /l/		
10/97	✓ in isolation		10/97
10/97	✓ in syllables	Probes to assess production in untrained contexts	10/97
11/97	✓ in words		11/97
12/97	✓ initial		12/97
1/98	✓ medial		1/98
2/98	✓ final		2/98
3/98	✓ in phrases		4/98
5/98	✓ in sentences		6/98
6/98	✓ conversational speech		not met
	✓ in natural settings		
6/98	increased intelligibility		partially met by 6/98

Gulf Coast Unified School District
Department of Special Educational Services
Language, Speech, and Hearing
Individualized Educational Program

TREATMENT OF VOICE DISORDERS

Student Name: _____   Speech-Language and Hearing Specialist

School: _____   _____

Program initiation date: _____   Date: _____

Goal: By <u>3/97</u>, the student will complete the following objectives with 80% accuracy.

Target Date	Objectives (Check the Ones Selected)	Evaluation and Treatment Procedures	Target Met On (Date)
	Voice Overall Objective: Improved voice quality and appropriate use of voice		
12/96	**Pitch** ✓ lower ___ higher ___ in school ___ in other settings	Successive approximation with the help of Visi-Pitch	12/96
12/96	**Intensity** ___ lower (softer voice) ✓ higher (louder voice) ___ in school ___ in other settings	Conversational probes to assess generalization and maintenance	12/96
	Nasal resonance ___ decrease ___ increase		
2/97 2/97 3/97	**Voice quality** ✓ reduce hoarseness ✓ reduce harshness ✓ reduce breathiness Other voice objectives (specify):		To be met

**North Central Unified School District
Speech, Language, and Hearing Services
Individualized Educational Plan**

TREATMENT OF FLUENCY DISORDERS

Student Name: _____   Speech-Language and Hearing Specialist

School: _____   _____

Treatment began on: _____   Date: _____

Goal: Improved fluency in conversational speech produced in extraclinical settings with a dysfluency rate under 5%.

Target Date	Objectives (Check the ones selected)	Evaluation and Treatment Procedures	Objectives Met On
	Fluency		
	Target Skills:	Teaching fluency skills with modeling, successive approximation, and verbal reinforcement.	
11/96	✓ Appropriate management of airflow	Fading the slow rate; shaping normal prosody	11/96
12/96	✓ Gentle phonatory onset		12/96
3/97	✓ Reduced rate of speech		3/97
4/97	✓ in words and phrases		Not met
5/97	✓ in sentences		Not met
5/97	✓ in conversational speech		Not met
6/97	✓ in extraclinical situations		Not met
	___ Normal prosody and fluency	Conversational probes to assess generalization to and maintenance of fluency in clinical and extraclinical situations	

Note to Student Clinicians

Contact the coordinator of speech-language and hearing services in one of the school districts in your area to learn more about variations in individualized educational plans written for students. Before you begin your clinical internships in a public school, practice writing individualized educational plans according to the format accepted in the school.

C.3. PRACTICE IN WRITING TREATMENT PLANS

On the following pages, you will find opportunities for you to practice writing treatment plans. Clinical data are given on the left-hand page. Use these data to write your treatment plans on the right-hand page.

You may wish to consult the corresponding exemplars in sections C.2.1 and C.2.2 before you write the reports in this section. Make sure that you vary your sentences.

Clinics vary in their format of treatment plans. The format used in this book does not include formally arranged identifying information that was included in assessment (diagnostic reports). However, if required by your clinic, you can place the identifying information at the beginning of the report in the following (or any other accepted) format:

TREATMENT PLAN

Client: **Birthdate:**

Address: **Clinic file number:**

City: **Date:**

Telephone number: **Diagnosis:**

Referred by: **Clinician:**

Supervisor:

C.3.1. COMPREHENSIVE TREATMENT PLAN: *LANGUAGE DISORDERS*

University Speech and Hearing Center
Pan Pacific University
Pacific, California

Data Sheet. Use these data to write your report on the opposite page. Use the correct headings.

Harvey Brokert, 6 years of age Talks in two-to-three-word phrases no sentences; no morphologic features	Background Information **(L1H)** Who, how old, when, to where referred? What were the results of evaluation? (Summarize the disorder) Was treatment recommended?
Treatment was recommended	
Mother will bring the child to treatment	
Good prognosis for improved language skills	
	Target Behaviors? **(L1H)**
Final target behaviors: Functional language skills with appropriate grammatic and pragmatic structures produced in natural settings	
Initial target behaviors: Teaching nouns, auxiliary *is* and verb + *ing; prepositions in, on* and *under;* and pronoun*s he* and *she.* All taught in the context of simple sentences	
Baserated on a set of modeled and evoked trials; 20 stimulus sentences for each target; baserates between 0 to 10%	

C.3.1. COMPREHENSIVE TREATMENT PLAN: *LANGUAGE DISORDERS*

Write your report. Use the information on the data sheet. Invent information as needed.

_____

_____

_____

_____

_____

_____

_____

_____

_____

_____

_____

_____

_____

_____

_____

_____

_____

_____

_____

_____

_____

_____

_____

_____

_____

Data Sheet. Use these data to write your report on the opposite page. Use the correct headings.

Discrete trial procedure:
    show the stimulus, ask a question, model the response,
    reinforce or give corrective feedback, record the response,
    re-present the stimulus for the next trial
	Treatment and
	Probe Procedures?
	(L1H)

Modeling, verbal praise, natural consequences Five consecutively and correctly imitated responses: shift to evoked Two incorrect responses on evoked trials: reinstate modeling	Various training and probe criteria
Training criterion: 10 consecutively correct, nonimitated responses for each target exemplar (phrase or sentence)	
Intermixed probe procedure: Will consist of trained and untrained sentences; trained responses will be reinforced, untrained responses will not be	
Correct probe response rate calculated based only on responses given to untrained (probe) stimuli	
Ninety percent correct probe response rate: shift training to another stimulus item, a more complex response topography, or another target behavior	
Not met the probe criterion, give more training on the same target behavior	
Eventually, train the target structures in conversational speech with social reinforcers	

Write your report. Use the information on the data sheet. Invent information as needed.

_____

_____

_____

_____

_____

_____

_____

_____

_____

_____

_____

_____

_____

_____

_____

_____

_____

_____

_____

_____

_____

_____

_____

_____

Data Sheet. Use these data to write your report on the opposite page. Use the correct headings.	
Training the mother in evoking and reinforcing the target language structures at home	Maintenance Program **(L1H)**
Initially, the mother observes sessions Then she learns to present stimulus items Then she learns to reinforce or give corrective feedback An older brother to be trained in reinforcing target responses	Training family members and others

Write your report. Use the information on the data sheet. Invent information as needed.

Data Sheet. Use these data to write your report on the opposite page. Use the correct headings.	
Informal training in nonclinical settings (specify a few settings)	Training in informal settings
Recorded home samples for probe analysis; 90% correct production at home is the maintenance criterion	Home samples
Additional training on other language structures to be determined later	Additional training
	Signature lines
	Student Clinician
	Client
	Supervisor
	Date

Write your report. Use the information on the data sheet. Invent information as needed.

C.3.2. BRIEF TREATMENT PLAN: *FLUENCY DISORDER*

Speech and Hearing Clinic
Eastern State University
Bedford, California

Data Sheet. Use these data to write your report on the opposite page. Use the correct headings.	
James Higginbothams, 27-year-old engineer Self-referred Two speech samples; 23% and 25% dysfluency rate in conversational speech (part-word repetitions, sound prolongations, word and phrase interjections, and broken words) Treatment was recommended Prognosis judged to be good because of expressed high motivation for treatment	Who, how old, when, to where referred? What were the results of evaluation? (Summarize the disorder.) Was treatment recommended?
Normal-sounding fluency with no more than 5% dysfluency rate in nonclinical settings	Final Treatment Objective?
Appropriate management of airflow (inhalation, a slight exhalation, sustained airflow), gentle phonatory onset, reduced speech rate with prolonged syllables, continuous phonation, and normal prosodic features	Target Behaviors? **(L1H)**

C.3.2. BRIEF TREATMENT PLAN: *FLUENCY DISORDER*

Write your report. Use the information on the data sheet. Invent information as needed.

_____

_____

_____

_____

_____

_____

_____

_____

_____

_____

_____

_____

_____

_____

_____

_____

_____

_____

_____

_____

_____

_____

_____

_____

_____

_____

_____

Data Sheet. Use these data to write your report on the opposite page. Use the correct headings.	
Initial baserating in conversational speech	Treatment Procedures? **(L1H)**
Training begins at phrase and short sentence levels	
Each target trained one at a time and then integrated	
Instructions and modeling	
Verbal reinforcement for the production of all target behaviors	
Corrective feedback for incorrect responses and dysfluencies	
Training of normal prosodic feature (when 2% or less dysfluency rate is sustained)	
Training wife and a colleague in fluency maintenance; training in extraclinical situations	
Training self monitoring skills	
Home speech samples to evaluate maintenance of fluency	
A schedule of follow-up; booster treatment	
	Signature lines
	Student Clinician
	Client
	Supervisor
	Date

Write your report. Use the information on the data sheet. Invent information as needed.

C.3.2. BRIEF TREATMENT PLAN: *ARTICULATION DISORDER*

Valley Speech and Hearing Center
Nordstrom, Maine

Data Sheet. Use these data to write your report on the opposite page. Use the correct headings.

Beth Hazleton, 9 years of age	Who, how old, when, to where referred? What were the results of evaluation? (Summarize the disorder.) Was treatment recommended?
Articulation disorder; omissions: (specify four to six phonemes); substitutions: (specify a few)	
Treatment recommended	
Mother to participate in treatment	
Ninety percent correct production in conversational speech in extraclinical situations	Final Treatment Objective? **(Paragraph heading)**
Objective 1. Correct production in all word positions (specify) with 90% accuracy	Objectives? Procedures? **(Paragraph headings)**
Procedures: Instructions, demonstrations, modeling, visual feedback, shaping, verbal reinforcement, corrective feedback	
Objective 2. Correct production in phrases and sentences	
Procedures: Picture description and controlled conversation; modeling, reinforcement, corrective feedback	

C.3.2. BRIEF TREATMENT PLAN: *ARTICULATION DISORDER*

Write your report. Use the information on the data sheet. Invent information as needed.

_____

_____

_____

_____

_____

_____

_____

_____

_____

_____

_____

_____

_____

_____

_____

_____

_____

_____

_____

_____

_____

_____

_____

_____

_____

_____

_____

	Paragraph headings for objectives and procedures
Data Sheet. Use these data to write your report on the opposite page. Use the correct headings.	
Objective 3. Correct production, conversational speech, varied audience	
Procedures: Reinforcement, varied audience	
Objective 4. Correct production in extraclinical situations	
Procedures: Prompting and reinforcing correct production in extraclinical settings (specify)	
Objective 5. Training the mother (in what?)	
Procedures: Initial observation, recognition of the target responses, reinforcement, home treatment sessions, taped home samples to be submitted	
Dismissal criterion, follow-up, booster treatment	
	Signature lines
	Student Clinician
	Parent
	Supervisor
	Date

Write your report. Use the information on the data sheet. Invent information as needed.

C.3.2. BRIEF TREATMENT PLAN: *LANGUAGE DISORDER*

Speech and Hearing Clinic
Southern State University
Johnstonville, Louisiana

Data Sheet. Use these data to write your report on the opposite page. Use the correct headings.

Harold Ford, 5 year old. Developmentally delayed Says only six to eight words No phrases, no sentences, no morphologic features Treatment was recommended	Who, how old, when, to where referred? What were the results of evaluation? (Summarize the disorder.) Was treatment recommended?
Correct production of 20 functional words or two-word phrases at 90% accuracy (invent words or phrases) Baserates: 5 to 10% correct	Initial Treatment Objectives? **Select a heading style**
Additional words Expansion of single words into phrases and sentences Morphological features (specify four)	Subsequent Treatment Objectives? **Repeat the selected heading style**

C.3.2. BRIEF TREATMENT PLAN: *LANGUAGE DISORDER*

Write your report. Use the information on the data sheet. Invent information as needed.

_____

_____

_____

_____

_____

_____

_____

_____

_____

_____

_____

_____

_____

_____

_____

_____

_____

_____

_____

_____

_____

Data Sheet. Use these data to write your report on the opposite page. Use the correct headings.	
Stimuli will include pictures and so forth (expand)	Initial Treatment Procedures? **Repeat the selected heading style**
Clinician and the mother to evoke the target language structures	
Initially, approximations accepted; subsequently, more accurate production	
Verbal praise and natural reinforcers	
Measurement of responses in each session	
Training criterion: 90% accuracy across two sessions for words; then an intermixed probe will be conducted	
Phrases formed out of words that meet the 90% accurate probe criterion	
Similar progression for sentences (describe)	
Home treatment sessions	
Taped home samples to monitor home treatment	
Subsequent Treatment Procedures	Subsequent Treatment Procedures **Repeat the selected heading style**
The same procedure described under initial treatment procedures	
Additional words expanded into phrases and sentences	
Teaching morphologic features initially in words and later expanded into phrases and sentences	
	Signature lines
	Student Clinician
	Client
	Supervisor
	Date

Write your report. Use the information on the data sheet. Invent information as needed.

C.3.2. BRIEF TREATMENT PLAN: *VOICE DISORDER*

The Sunshine Speech and Hearing Center
Zingsville, Vermont

Data Sheet. Use these data to write your report on the opposite page. Use the correct headings.

Thomas Benson, Jr., 28 years of age	Who, how old, when, to where referred? What were the results of evaluation? (Summarize the disorder.) Was treatment recommended?
Long history of high-pitched voice	
Laryngologist has cleared for voice treatment	
Treatment was recommended	
	Use the format given in C.2.2. Brief Treatment Plan: Voice Disorders
Treatment Targets	
Vocal pitch judged appropriate for age and gender	**Select a heading style and use it consistently**
Lowered pitch level in words, phrases, sentences, and conversational speech (write them as separate goals)	

C.3.2. BRIEF TREATMENT PLAN: *VOICE DISORDER*

Write your report. Use the information on the data sheet. Invent information as needed.

Data Sheet. Use these data to write your report on the opposite page. Use the correct headings.	
Shaping lower-pitched voice through modeling and verbal feedback Starting with words and progressing to conversational speech Other procedures you select	Treatment Procedures **Use the selected heading style**
Ninety percent accuracy at each level of training Ninety percent probe criterion in natural settings Home samples to monitor voice at home	
Self-monitoring skills	Training family members and others
Training Ms. Moline Benson (the client's wife) in monitoring and reinforcing appropriate pitch at home; informal home treatment sessions	
Home sample to evaluate the home treatment sessions	Signature lines
Standard follow-up and booster treatment	Student Clinician Supervisor Client Date

Write your report. Use the information on the data sheet. Invent information as needed.

_____

_____

_____

_____

_____

_____

_____

_____

_____

_____

_____

_____

_____

_____

_____

_____

_____

_____

_____

_____

_____

_____

_____

_____

_____

_____

Note to Student Clinicians

Clinical supervisors tend to have their preferred formats for writing treatment plans. Talk to your supervisor before you write treatment plans for your clients.

C.4. PROGRESS REPORTS

Progress reports summarize the methods and results of treatment given during a specified period of time. In academic degree programs, progress reports are typically written at the end of a quarter or semester. In some university programs, progress reports also may be known as *final summaries*. In hospitals and private clinics, they are written according to a setting-specific policy. Generally, insurance companies and government or private agencies require them to support payment for services. In such cases, they may be written on a monthly basis. Progress reports are written invariably when the clients are dismissed from services.

Progress reports students write under clinical practicum or internship is more likely to give such additional information as the number of and duration of sessions and the clock hours of clinical practicum. Such information is not a part of reports professional clinicians write.

Most progress reports are formal documents written for the file. In some settings, especially in hospitals and private clinics, progress reports may be written in the form of a letter to a referring physician or to a funding agency.

Formats used for progress reports vary across clinics. The reports that follow in this section show a few variations. For example, the first report on fluency disorder refers the reader to a treatment plan in the folder, and therefore, does not summarize the procedures. Whereas, the next report on an articulation disorder makes no mention of a treatment plan; instead, it summarizes the procedures and results (progress).

The student clinicians should consult their clinic director or clinical supervisor to find out the format adopted for the clinic or setting.

C.4. PROGRESS REPORT: TREATMENT OF *STUTTERING*

University Speech and Hearing Clinic
Freemont University
Valleyville, California

PROGRESS REPORT

NAME: James Foxx

BIRTHDATE: January xx, xxxx

ADDRESS: Graves 312 B

CITY: Valleyville, CA 90710-3342

TELEPHONE NUMBER: 555-3235

FILE NUMBER: RS92019

DIAGNOSIS: Stuttering

DATE OF REPORT: May xx, xxxx

PERIOD COVERED: xx/xx/xx to xx-xx-xx

CLINICIAN: Meena Wong

CLINIC SCHEDULE

Session per week: 2
Length of session: 50 min
Number of clinic visits: 24

Clock hrs of individual therapy: 25
Clock hrs of group therapy: 0
Total clock hrs. of therapy: 25

James Foxx, a 21-year-old male college student, was enrolled for his first semester of treatment at the University Speech and Hearing Clinic on February xx, xxxx. The presenting complaint was stuttering. An assessment done on February x, xxxx had revealed a conversational dysfluency rate of 21% in the clinic. A home speech sample had revealed a dysfluency rate of 18.6%. He exhibited interjections, pauses, part-word and whole-word repetitions, silent and audible prolongations, revisions, and incomplete phrases.

Treatment was begun on February 5, 1992. An assessment report may be found in Mr. Foxx's folder.

SUMMARY OF TREATMENT

Final Treatment Objective: Maintenance of fluent speech with a dysfluency rate that does not exceed 5% in natural settings.

TARGET BEHAVIORS

Fluency skills described in the treatment plan were taught: Appropriate management of airflow, gentle onset of phonation, reduced speech rate, continuos phonation, and normal prosodic features. Please see Mr. Foxx's file for his treatment plan for details.

TREATMENT PROCEDURES

In two clinic baseline samples of conversational speech and a home baseline sample, Mr. Foxx's dysfluency rates were 22%, 21%, and 19%.

Initially, Mr. Foxx was taught the skills of fluent speech: nasal inhalation, minimal amount of oral exhalation prior to initiation of phonation, easy phonatory onset, and vowel prolongation. Therapy was started at the modeled word level and progressed to words, phrases, sentences, and conversational speech in the clinic. At each level, 98% fluency was required. Verbal reinforcement was provided on an FR1 schedule. Corrective feedback was given for dysfluencies or failure to manage a target behavior. Mr. Foxx was then required to correctly repeat his utterance.

After Mr. Foxx had progressed to conversational speech, he was taught to chart his dysfluencies and failure to use a target behavior. Periodically, Mr. Foxx orally read printed stories and then summarized what he had read. Student observers periodically participated in treatment sessions to engage in conversation with the client.

Normal prosodic features were not targeted this semester, as the establishment of stutter-free speech was not completed.

Mr. Foxx's wife attended four treatment sessions and a colleague of his attended 2 sessions. Both were trained in prompting Mr. Foxx to use the fluency skills and to reinforce him.

PROGRESS

Two clinic probes and a home probe were obtained after the client began using the target fluency skills in conversational speech in the clinic (probes #1 and #2). Each probe consisted of 50 utterances sampled from the client's conversational speech. The results were as follows.

Probe #1: 15% dysfluent (Clinic Sample)

Probe #2: 12% dysfluent (Clinic Sample)

Probe #3: 10% dysfluent (Home Sample)

A final conversational speech sample containing 852 words in 102 utterances was obtained in the semester's final treatment session. This sample was obtained through a conversation with a student observer in the absence of the clinician. Results were as follows:

Dysfluency Types	Frequency
Interjections	23
Pauses	17
Part Word Repetitions	1
Whole Word Repetitions	3
Phrase Repetitions	2
Sound Prolongations	20
Silent Prolongations	6
Incomplete Phrases	2
Total Dysfluencies	**74**
Percent Dysfluency Rate	**8.9**

The results show that Mr. Foxx's fluency improved over the course of the semester. He was about 21% dysfluent at the beginning of treatment compared to 8.9% dysfluent at the end of the semester.

RECOMMENDATIONS

Although Mr. Foxx's dysfluencies have decreased, he continues to exhibit difficulty in consistently managing the target behaviors. Therefore, it is recommended that Mr. Foxx continue to receive treatment next semester. The clinician should concentrate on the following:

1. Improved management of fluency skills
2. Generalization and maintenance of fluent speech

Submitted by:_____

      Layang Chan, B.A.
      Student Clinician

Client's or Parents' Signature:_____

      Mr. James Foxx

Approved by:_____

      Linda Hensley, Ph.D., CCC-SLP
      Speech-Language Pathologist and Clinical Supervisor

Date:_____

| **C.4. PROGRESS REPORT: TREATMENT OF AN *ARTICULATION DISORDER*** |

Speech and Hearing Center
Henry Higgins Children's Hospital
Burlington, Vermont

PROGRESS REPORT

Period Covered: xx/xx/xx to xx/xx/xx

Background Information

Joe Villa, a 6-year and 3-month-old boy, was seen for a speech and language evaluation at the Speech and Hearing Center of the Henry Higgins Children's Hospital on September xx, xxxx. Joe has an articulation disorder characterized mostly by omissions of /s/, /t/, /k/, /b/, and /l/ in the initial and final position of words. An articulation treatment program was recommended. He has received treatment at this facility for 4 months.

The final treatment objective for Joe was to produce the phonemes he omits with 90% accuracy in conversational speech in extraclinical situations.

PROGRESS

Objective 1. Correct production of /s/, /t/, /k/, /b/, and /l/ in word initial positions with 90% accuracy.

Method and Results: The target phoneme production in word initial positions was baserated on a set of modeled and evoked trials with 20 words for each phoneme. Joe's correct response rate ranged from 0 to 10%. Treatment was begun with the discrete trial procedure involving modeling, imitation, successive approximation, and immediate verbal feedback for correct and incorrect responses. Whenever necessary, the tongue positions were shown with the help of a mirror. Each target sound was trained to a criterion of 10 consecutively correct responses. When four words with a target sound met the training criterion, at least 10 probe words were presented to assess generalization.

Joe has met this training objective. His correct response rates on these phonemes in word initial positions varied between 95 and 100%.

Objective 2. Correct production of /s/, /t/, /k/, /b/, and /l/ in word final positions with 90% accuracy.

Methods and Results: The same procedures used to train the phonemes in the word initial positions were used. Joe has met this objective. His correct response rates on the phonemes in word final positions varied between 92 and 96%.

Objective 3. Production of the target sounds in phrases and sentences with 90% accuracy in all word positions.

Methods and Results: Joe's correct productions were initially reinforced in phrases that were prepared for training. Soon, he was asked to use the target words in sentences he formulated. Later, Joe's conversational speech was monitored to strengthen the correct production of the phonemes. Verbal reinforcement was used on an FR4 schedule.

Joe has met this objective as his correct production of the target phonemes in conversational speech varied between 90 and 95%.

Objective 4. The development and implementation of a home program to maintain the production of his new speech skills in natural settings with 90% accuracy.

Methods and Results: Joe's parents, who attended most of the treatment sessions, were trained to recognize, prompt, and reinforce the correct production of target sounds. Parents were asked to hold home treatment sessions twice a week and tape-record the sessions. These taped samples were analyzed to give feedback to the parents. Three conversational probes recorded at home have revealed a 90% correct response rate.

Overall, Joe has made excellent progress in producing the targeted sounds. All treatment objective have been met. Therefore, it is recommended that Joe be dismissed from treatment. A follow-up assessment in 3 months is recommended.

Monica Mendoza, M.A., CCC-SLP
Speech-Language Pathologist

C.4. PROGRESS REPORT: *LANGUAGE TREATMENT*

**University Speech and Hearing Center
Bellview University
Bellview, Washington**

Client: William Shakespeare

Date of Birth: January xx, xxx

Period Covered: xx/xx through xx/xx, xxxx

Clinician: Noah Webster

CLINIC SCHEDULE

Session per week: 2
Length of session: 40 min
Number of clinic visits: 24

Clock hr of individual therapy: 25
Clock hr of group therapy: 0
Total clock hr of therapy: 25

William Shakespeare, a 7-year-old boy, was assessed at the University Speech and Hearing Center of Bellview University for a language disorder. The assessment suggested that his language disorder primarily involved some syntactic structures and pragmatic functions. Treatment was recommended. He has received treatment for one semester. Please see his clinic file for an assessment report and a complete treatment program.

SUMMARY OF TREATMENT

William was cooperative in most treatment sessions. The following treatment procedures and objectives were used.

Objective 1. Asking *WH* Questions

William was taught to ask the following types of *wh* questions:

What do you mean?

What is it?

What are you doing?

What time is it?

What is your name?

Methods and Results: Baserating showed that William typically did not ask the target questions even when the situation demanded them. In a conversational role-playing situation, William was taught to ask the target questions. Conversational situations were created such that questions of the kind targeted would be appropriate. Conversation was manipulated in various ways to prompt the a target question. For example, William was asked, "Do you live in a condo?" and was immediately modeled the correct question for him to imitate: "William, ask me *what do you mean?*" Or, he was shown a picture he did not know anything about and immediately the question "What is it?" was modeled for him to imitate. When William imitated modeled questions or asked similar questions without modeling, the clinician correctly answered them. These answers and verbal praise for asking appropriate questions were the reinforcers.

When William; question-asking reached 90% accuracy, probes were conducted to assess generalized question-asking. The probe results showed that William learned to ask the targeted questions in untrained (probe) contexts with 90% accuracy.

Objective 2. Topic Maintenance

William was taught to maintain a topic of conversation for progressively increasing durations with 90% accuracy.

Methods and Results: Baserating showed that William typically changed the topic in less than a min. He was taught to maintain a topic of conversation for progressively longer durations. One-minute increments were used. Starting with a duration of 1 min, he was taught to talk about the same topic for a maximum duration of 5 min. Every time he deviated from the topic, the clinician asked him to stop and prompted him to resume the target topic. He was periodically praised for continuing on the same topic.

William learned to maintain a topic of conversation for a minimum of 5 min. On certain probe topics, he continued to talk for up to 10 min.

Objective 3. Conversational Turn Taking

William was taught to take appropriate conversational turns with 90% accuracy.

Methods and Results: During the baserating, William typically interrupted the clinician every 30 sec. He was initially asked to speak only when told, "It is your turn to talk." Clinician gave William his turn every 1 min or so. William also was taught to say, "It is your turn to talk," when he had spoken for a minute or so. If he did not, he was asked to stop at the end of a sentence. The prompt, "It is your turn to talk," was withdrawn in the latter training sessions. If he interrupted, the clinician gave a hand signal to stop. This signal also was faded. In the last four sessions, a variable time interval of 1 to 3 min of talking before yielding the floor was allowed.

William learned to take conversational turns. On a final probe with no verbal or manual prompt, he took turns on the variable time schedule of 1 to 3 minutes of talking with 90% accuracy. Occasionally, he appropriately exceeded the range.

A final spontaneous language sample was analyzed to determine the need for further clinical services. The analysis revealed an essentially normal language use. Therefore, it is recommended that William be dismissed from treatment.

_____
Noah Webster, B.A.
Student Clinician

_____
Mrs. Tara Shakespeare
Parent

_____
Lakshmi Shanker, Ph.D., CCC-SLP
Speech-Language Pathologist and Clinical Supervisor

Date:_____

C.4. PROGRESS REPORT: *VOICE TREATMENT*

Siera Speech and Hearing Center
Clovis, CA

PROGRESS REPORT

NAME: Roshana Hersh	**FILE NUMBER:** Axxcqxxx
BIRTHDATE: January xx, xxxx	**DIAGNOSIS:** Voice Disorder
ADDRESS: 7915 Vishon	**DATE OF REPORT:** February xx, xxxx
CITY: Clovis, CA 93611	**PERIOD COVERED:** September xx through December xx, xxxx
TELEPHONE NUMBER:	**CLINICIAN:** Pero Boss **Supervisor:** Moss Nero, M.A., CCC-SLP

Roshana Hersh, a 21-year-old female college student, was seen at the Sierra Speech and Hearing Center on September xx, xxxx for a voice evaluation. The evaluation suggested a pattern of vocal abuse associated with a persistent hoarseness of voice and low pitch. A treatment program to improve her voice quality was recommended. The assessment report and a description of her treatment program may be found in her clinical file.

TREATMENT TARGETS

Goal 1: Production of clear voice at least 90% of the time Roshana speaks by reducing the hoarseness of voice
    Objective 1a. Reduced amount of talking over the phone.
    Objective 1b. Reduced amount of shouting at the school.
Goal 2: Increased vocal pitch
    Objective 2a. Higher pitch at the level of words and phrases.
    Objective 2b. Higher pitch at the level of conversational speech.

TREATMENT PROCEDURES AND RESULTS

Objectives 1a and 1b. During the first week, the durations of Ms. Hersh's telephone conversation were baserated. The diary record she kept showed that Roshana spoke between 8 to 10 times over the phone each day and that the duration of her phone calls ranged between 10 to 20 min. Sixty percent of her phone calls typically exceeded 15 min.

During the second week, Ms. Hersh was asked to reduce by 10% the amount of telephone conversation time. She continued to record the amount of time she spent talking over the phone. In subsequent weeks, she was asked to progressively decrease the amount of time spent on the telephone with a goal of reducing the duration by about 50%.

The frequency of shouting also was similarly baserated. On an average day, she tended to shout 8 to 10 times. Ms. Hersh was asked to reduce the frequency of shouting behavior in 10% decrements until the frequency approached zero.

Ms. Hersh made excellent progress in reducing the frequency and duration of phone calls and in reducing the frequency of shouting. At the end of the semester, her phone calls averaged between 3 to 7 min. Only an exceptional phone call exceeded this range. Her shouting behavior was reduced to no more than two incidents per day. According to Ms. Hersh, her shouts are not as loud as they used to be.

Objectives 2a and 2b. The Visi-Pitch was used to shape a higher pitch consistent with Ms. Hersh's gender and age. The treatment was started at the word and phrase level and moved to conversational speech level.

Ms. Hersh's speaking fundamental frequency in the clinic increased from a baserate of 157 Hz to 200 Hz toward the end of the semester. However, she still reports a much lower pitch outside the clinic.

It is recommended that Ms. Hersh continue to receive voice therapy next semester. The emphasis should be on generalization and maintenance of appropriate target vocal characteristics in extraclinical situations. Ms. Hersh needs training in self-monitoring skills.

Signed:_____
      Pero Boss, B.A.
      Student Clinician

Signed:_____
      Ms. Roshana Hersh

Signed:_____
      Moss Nero, M.A., CCC-SLP
      Speech-Language Pathologist and Clinical Supervisor

Date:_____

Note to Student Clinicians

Contact your clinic director to find out how progress reports vary in your clinic. Contact a private speech and hearing clinic to find out how clinicians there write progress reports they send to health insurance companies.

C.4.1. PROGRESS REPORTS WRITTEN AS LETTERS

Some progress reports are written in the form of a letter. Such progress reports are necessary when clinicians:

- make a referral to another professional for continued speech-language services
- make a referral to a different professional
- make a claim for payment for services from an agency

C.4.1. PROGRESS REPORT: *WRITTEN AS A LETTER*

Southern California Speech and Hearing Center
Long Beach, California

April xx, xxxx

Dr. Kim Yang
Long Beach Neurologists, Inc.
Long Beach, California

RE: Juniper Joginder

Dear Dr. Yang:

I am referring Mr. Joginder, a 57-year-old man, to you for a neurological examination. Mr. Joginder experienced a left hemisphere CVA on February 7, xxxx, and was subsequently admitted to St. Thomas Medical Center. On February 12, xxxx, he was transferred to Los Angeles Rehabilitation Hospital (LARH) where he received physical therapy, occupational therapy, and speech therapy. A speech-language evaluation was completed at LARH. Mr. Joginder was diagnosed with severe receptive and expressive aphasia and severe apraxia of speech. He received speech-language therapy at LARH from February 12, xxxx, to May 31, xxxx. The staff at LARH has documented Mr. Joginder's level of functioning while he was at that facility, and you may obtain their report for details. Upon his discharge from LARH, Mr. Joginder began receiving speech-language therapy at Southern California Speech and Hearing Center. He has attended therapy twice a week for a total of 60 visits.

Initially, Mr. Joginder's understanding of spoken speech and reading were moderately impaired. These skills are now within normal limits and completely functional.

Mr. Joginder's expressive language was severely impaired. Following the CVA, he was virtually non-verbal except for a few paraphasic utterances. Word retrieval deficits and verbal apraxia were severe. When he began therapy at Southern California Speech and Hearing Center, Mr. Joginder was working on word retrieval, producing multisyllable words (90%), and using multisyllable words in a variety of target sentence structures (70%). His word retrieval skills have improved significantly. He currently can cite antonyms or synonyms with 90 to 100% accuracy, provide words when given a description or definition with 90% accuracy, and name pictures with 90 to 100% accuracy. Mr. Joginder can formulate sentences when given a word with 70 to 90% accuracy, answer simple questions with 80 to 90% accuracy, and describe pictures with 90 to 100% accuracy.

Most recently, I have been working with Mr. Joginderís lecture notes. Currently, he can organize and create a written outline on his own. Using his outline, he can now present a 30 to 45 min lecture with 75 to 90% accuracy. He can answer simple questions about the lecture with 70 to 80% accuracy.

Overall, Mr. Joginder has made remarkable progress in all targeted speech-language skills. He has excellent family support. Therefore, it is recommended that he continue to receive speech-language therapy with an emphasis on:

1. high-level word retrieval skills
2. sentence and question formulation
3. spontaneous responses to questions
4. lecturing skills
5. accurate production of his work-related vocabulary
6. accurate production of multi-syllable words and words containing difficult blends or sound combinations, and
7. overall conversational speech skills

I hope this information is helpful. I look forward to receiving your report on Mr. Joginder. Please contact me if you have questions. Thank you.

Yours sincerely,

_____

Von Tran, M.A., CCC-SLP
Speech-Language Pathologist

Date:_____

Note to Student Clinicians

Contact your supervisor and directors of private speech clinics to find out what kinds of letters are typically sent to government agencies that reimburse clinicians for speech, language, and hearing services. Some agencies may use printed forms. Obtain samples of such forms.

C.5. PRACTICE IN WRITING PROGRESS REPORTS

C.5. PROGRESS REPORT: TREATMENT OF *STUTTERING*

University Speech and Hearing Clinic
Freemont University
Valleyville, California

PROGRESS REPORT

Name: Winston Churchill

Birthdate:

Address:

City:

Telephone number:

File number:

Diagnosis: Stuttering

Date of report:

Period covered:

Clinician:

CLINIC SCHEDULE

Sessions per week:

Length of sessions:

Number of clinic visits:

Clock hr of individual therapy:

Clock hr of group therapy:

Total clock hr of therapy:

Data Sheet. Use these data to write your report on the opposite page. Use the correct headings.

Winston Churchill, 22 years of age	Who, how old, came to which clinic, and with what problem?
Stuttering since early childhood days; various ineffective treatments in the past	
Two conversational speech samples (9 and 11% dysfluency rate)	(Summarize the assessment data in one or two sentences.)
One reading sample (22% dysfluency rate)	
Received treatment for stuttering for one semester at the same facility; the same treatment as described next	Received treatment for what and for how long?

C.5. PROGRESS REPORT: TREATMENT OF *STUTTERING*

Write your report. Use the information on the data sheet. Invent information as needed.

_____

_____

_____

_____

_____

_____

_____

_____

_____

_____

_____

_____

_____

_____

_____

_____

_____

_____

_____

_____

_____

_____

_____

_____

_____

_____

Data Sheet. Use these data to write your report on the opposite page. Use the correct headings.

Final Treatment Goal: Normal-sounding fluency in natural settings with less than 5% dysfluency rate (or any other objectives you select)	**Select a heading style and use it consistently**
Two conversational speech baselines of 10 and 11% dysfluency or stuttering rate	Baselines
Airflow management (specify the components) Gentle phonatory onset Continuous phonation Rate reduction through syllable stretching Normal prosodic features	Treatment Targets
Modeling and imitation; controlled utterances; movement from words to phrases and conversational speech; verbal praise; corrective feedback for mismanagement of the target behaviors or for dysfluencies; 98% or better fluency at all stages; periodic probes with no treatment contingencies to assess generalized fluency; twice-a-week sessions of 50 minutes; dysfluencies and errors in target skills measured in all sessions	Treatment, probe, and measurement procedures.
Roommate trained in prompting and reinforcing the production of fluency skills in three treatment sessions	

Write your report. Use the information on the data sheet. Invent information as needed.

_____

_____

_____

_____

_____

_____

_____

_____

_____

_____

_____

_____

_____

_____

_____

_____

_____

_____

_____

_____

_____

_____

_____

_____

_____

_____

Data Sheet. Use these data to write your report on the opposite page. Use the correct headings.

Results or Progress

Good progress: Dysfluency rates reduced to 5% in conversational probes in the clinic (two probe conversational speech samples); about 6 to 7% at home (one home speech sample)

Continued treatment recommended to further reduce the dysfluencies and to stabilize fluency in naturalistic settings through informal treatment in various nonclinical settings (specify a few)

Continue with the selected heading style

What were the results?
Recommendations

Signature lines

Student Clinician

Client

Supervisor

Date

Write your report. Use the information on the data sheet. Invent information as needed.

C.5. PROGRESS REPORT: TREATMENT OF AN *ARTICULATION DISORDER*

University Speech and Hearing Center
Bloom, Illinois
PROGRESS REPORT

Name: Jimmy Jones   File number:

Birthdate: Diagnosis: Articulation disorder

Address: Date of report:

City: Period covered:

Telephone number: Clinician:

CLINIC SCHEDULE

Sessions per week: Clock hr of individual therapy:

Length of sessions: Clock hr of group therapy:

Number of clinic visits: Total clock hr of therapy:

Data Sheet. Use these data to write your report on the opposite page. Use the correct headings.

Jimmy Jones, 6 years of age

Articulation disorder
Omissions of initial and final /k, s, t, p, b/

No prior treatment

Select a heading style and use it consistently

Who, how old, came to which clinic and with what problem?

Summarize the assessment data in one or two sentences.

Received treatment for what and for how long?

C.5. PROGRESS REPORT: TREATMENT OF AN *ARTICULATION DISORDER*

Write your report. Use the information on the data sheet. Invent information as needed.

Data Sheet. Use these data to write your report on the opposite page. Use the correct headings.

Treatment Objective 1: Teaching the phonemes in word initial and final positions

Baserated: 0 to 5% correct response rate on evoked; 5 to 10% correct response rate on modeled trials

Treatment Procedures: Modeling, imitation, successive approximation, visual feedback (phonetic placement); positive reinforcement for correct responses and corrective feedback for wrong responses

Training criterion (90% correct) for any phoneme in any position
Probe criterion: 95% correct (intermixed probe: trained and untrained words; reinforcement only for the trained words)

Met the probe criterion for initial and final positions

Production of phonemes in phrases and sentences
Probe: 95% correct

Treatment Objective 2: Production of target phonemes in phrases and sentences

The same training and probe criteria (specify)

Met the probe criterion for phrases and sentences

Treatment Objective 3: Production of target phonemes in conversational speech

The same training and probe criteria (specify)

Did not meet the probe criterion (showed only 70% correct in conversational speech)

Continue with the selected heading style

Progress or Methods and Results

Write your report. Use the information on the data sheet. Invent information as needed.

Data Sheet. Use these data to write your report on the opposite page. Use the correct headings.

	Continue with the selected heading style
Development of a home treatment program for maintenance	Maintenance program
Training the father in evoking and reinforcing the phonemes in conversational speech at home	
Additional treatment to obtain and stabilize correct productions in conversational speech at 90% accuracy	Recommendations
	Signature lines
Your name	Student Clinician
The Client's Father's Name	Parent
Your Supervisor's name	Supervisor
Date	Date

Write your report. Use the information on the data sheet. Invent information as needed.

C.5. PROGRESS REPORT: TREATMENT OF *LANGUAGE DISORDER*

University Speech and Hearing Center
Bellview University
Bellview, Washington

PROGRESS REPORT

Name: Tanya Tucker   **File number:**
Birthdate: **Diagnosis: Language Disorder**
Address: **Date of report:**
City: **Period covered:**
Telephone number: **Clinician:**

CLINIC SCHEDULE

Sessions per week: **Clock hr of individual therapy:**
Length of sessions: **Clock hr of group therapy:**
Number of clinic visits: **Total clock hr of therapy:**

Data Sheet. Use these data to write your report on the opposite page. Use the correct headings.

Tanya Tucker, 6 years of age

Language disorders. Does not produce *ing*, auxiliary *is*, regular and irregular plurals, regular past tense, prepositions, and pronouns

Two semesters of treatment on teaching functional words and expansion of words into phrases; has met most probe criteria on these

Select a heading style and use it consistently

Who, how old, came to which clinic, and with what problem?

Summarize the assessment data in one or two sentences.

Received treatment for what and for how long?

C.5. PROGRESS REPORT: TREATMENT OF *LANGUAGE DISORDER*

Write your report. Use the information on the data sheet. Invent information as needed.

Data Sheet. Use these data to write your report on the opposite page. Use the correct headings.

Treatment Targets: Present progressive *ing*, auxiliary *is*, and regular plural morpheme *s* (e.g., *books* and *cups*) in sentences during the current semester of treatment	**Use the selected heading style consistently**
Pictures to evoke the target structures	
Training criterion: Ninety percent correct in words, phrases, and sentences	
Probe criterion: Ninety percent correct on a set of 10 untrained words, and untrained words used in phrases and sentences	
Twenty words, phrases, and sentences for each target. Baserate: 0 to 10% correct	
Discrete trial training at the level of words, phrases, and sentences	
Treatment procedures included stimulus presentation, appropriate question asking, modeling, reinforcement, and correct feedback	

Write your report. Use the information on the data sheet. Invent information as needed.

_____
_____
_____
_____
_____
_____
_____
_____
_____
_____
_____
_____
_____
_____
_____
_____
_____
_____
_____
_____
_____
_____

> Data Sheet. Use these data to write your report on the opposite page. Use the correct headings.

Results or Progress

Tanya made good progress in learning the language structures

Met the probe criteria for words and phrases for all targets

For sentences: Present progressive *ing*: Eight sentences trained; probe response rate: 90% correct probe response rate (thus has met the probe criterion)

Auxiliary *is*: Six sentences trained; 70% correct probe response rate

Regular plural s morpheme: four sentences trained; 80% correct probe response rate

Mother has received training in evoking and reinforcing the target structures at home

A home sample showed: 87% correct for the *ing*; 65% for the auxiliary *is*; and 70% for the plural *s*

Recommendations:

Continued treatment on the auxiliary and the plural morpheme to meet the probe criterion

Training to be shifted to conversational speech level for the present progressive *ing*

Training on additional grammatic morphemes Tanya does not produce

Continue to promote home training

Your name

Parent's name

Your supervisor's name

Date

Use the selected heading style consistently
Signature lines
Student Clinician
Parent
Supervisor
Date

Write your report. Use the information on the data sheet. Invent information as needed.

_____

_____

_____

_____

_____

_____

_____

_____

_____

_____

_____

_____

_____

_____

_____

_____

_____

_____

_____

_____

_____

_____

_____

_____

_____

_____

> ## C.5. PROGRESS REPORT: *VOICE DISORDER*

The Sunshine Speech and Hearing Center
Zingsville, Vermont

PROGRESS REPORT

Name: Raj Mohan

Birthdate:

Address:

City:

Telephone number:

File number:

Diagnosis: Voice disorder

Date of report:

Period covered:

Clinician:

CLINIC SCHEDULE

Sessions per week:

Length of sessions:

Number of clinic visits:

Clock hr of individual therapy:

Clock hr of group therapy:

Total clock hr of therapy:

Data Sheet. Use these data to write your report on the opposite page. Use the correct headings.

Raj Mohan, 35 years of age
High school teacher

| Select a heading style and use it consistently |

Inadequate loudness; voice too soft; students complain; his voice gets tired; ENT report negative; no contraindications for voice therapy

No prior treatment

C.5. PROGRESS REPORT: *VOICE DISORDER*

Write your report. Use the information on the data sheet. Invent information as needed.

_____

_____

_____

_____

_____

_____

_____

_____

_____

_____

_____

_____

_____

_____

_____

_____

_____

_____

_____

_____

_____

_____

_____

_____

_____

Data Sheet. Use these data to write your report on the opposite page. Use the correct headings.	
Treatment Targets: Increased vocal loudness; adequate loudness for classroom teaching as rated by the clinician and his students across a minimum of four teaching sessions Baseline of loudness established by: The clinician's and students' rating of loudness on a 5-point rating scale in three class periods Recording the frequency of student requests for louder speech (invent baseline data) Treatment Procedures Included verbal reinforcement of progressively louder speech Masking noise to increase vocal intensity (Lombard effect) Visi-Pitch feedback to shape progressively louder voice	**Use the selected heading style consistently**

Write your report. Use the information on the data sheet. Invent information as needed.

Data Sheet. Use these data to write your report on the opposite page. Use the correct headings.

	Use the selected heading style consistently
Results or Progress	
Excellent progress; Clinician's rating of loudness in three class periods showed adequate loudness; no student request for louder speech in the three observed class periods (compare this to baseline data)	
Schedule a follow-up in 3 months to assess maintenance of adequate loudness	
Recommendations: Dismissal from treatment; 3 and 6 month follow-up and booster treatment if necessary	
Your name	Student Clinician
Client's name	Client
Supervisor's name	Supervisor
Date	Date

Write your report. Use the information on the data sheet. Invent information as needed.

_____

_____

_____

_____

_____

_____

_____

_____

_____

_____

_____

_____

_____

_____

_____

_____

_____

_____

_____

_____

_____

_____

_____

_____

_____

C.5.1. PROGRESS REPORT: *WRITTEN AS A LETTER*

On the next page, write a letter to a speech-language pathologist (SLP) describing *the progress a 7-year-old boy with an articulation disorder* made under your treatment. Invent information as needed. The reason for referral: The child's family is moving to a new town and the SLP receiving the letter is expected to treat the child.

Data Sheet. Use these data to write your report on the opposite page. Use the correct headings.

The name of your Clinic

Date

Describe the child and his problems

Give a brief history

Summarize your assessment: Conversational speech sample and Goldman Fristoe Test of Articulation; the boy misarticulated six speech sounds (invent)

Summarize your treatment targets or objectives

Summarize your treatment procedures

Summarize the results or the progress (good progress; correct production of four phonemes in conversational speech; two more in need of treatment)

State your recommendations

Write your name, degree, and the CCC-SLP

Sign your name

C.5.1. PROGRESS REPORT: *WRITTEN AS A LETTER*

Write your letter. Invent information as needed. Use a standard letter format.

_____

_____

_____

_____

_____

_____

_____

_____

_____

_____

_____

_____

_____

_____

_____

_____

_____

_____

_____

_____

_____

Note to Student Clinicians

Obtain samples of progress reports from your clinic director. Practice writing reports on other disorders of communication.

C.6. PROFESSIONAL CORRESPONDENCE

Correspondence with clients, parents of clients, teachers, medical and other specialists is an important part of clinical duties. The letters a professional person writes about his or her services reflect training and competence. A well written letter may inspire confidence in a clinician, whereas a clumsy letter may detract potential clients or referrals. Professional letters should look good as well. This means that they should be on a letterhead printed on 25% cotton bond paper.

Professional letters should be:

- Accurate
    Give correct information based only on your observations.
- Brief and to the point
    Those who receive your letter may be busy people. So be brief and give only the most essential information.
- Suitable to the person receiving it
    If you write a letter to another professional who is expected to know your technical terms, use those terms. If the recipient is expected not to know your technical terms, use general terms.

Professional letters also include:

- *Thank you* letters written to persons or agencies that referred a client.
- Letters that describe treatment progress (usually sent to a referring or paying agency).
- Letters that make a referral to another professional.

C.6.I. A *THANK YOU* LETTER

California State University, Fresno
Speech and Hearing Clinic
Fresno, CA 93740

September x, xxxx

Dr. John Lamp
Lamp Pediatric Medical Group
4005 E. Marks
Fresno, CA 93728

Dear Dr. Lamp:

Thank you for referring Eric Martinez to the Speech and Hearing Clinic at California State University, Fresno for stuttering evaluation and treatment. We evaluated Eric's speech and language on September x, xxxx. Eric's mother brought him to the clinic. Mrs. Martinez brought a tape recorded speech sample from home which was analyzed as part of the evaluation.

Results of the assessment revealed a moderate to severe stuttering with a dysfluency rate of 15 to 20%. His stuttering is characterized by sound repetitions, intralexical pauses, interjections, and pauses. A few articulation errors were noted but did not interfere with speech intelligibility. Receptive and expressive language were judged age-appropriate.

It was recommended that Eric receive treatment for his stuttering. He is currently enrolled at the CSUF Speech and Hearing Clinic. In December, we will let you know about Eric's progress in treatment. If you have questions, please contact the clinic at 555-2142.

Sincerely,

_____
Athena Bacona, B.A.
Student Clinician

_____
Winthrop Venkat, M.A., CCC-SLP
Supervisor, Speech-Language Pathologist

C.6.2. A *REFERRAL* LETTER

Sunshine Speech and Hearing Clinic
Sunshine, MN

September xx, xxxx

Kristen Goodnow, M.D.
25 E. Cloudy, Suite 301
Sunshine, MN 00501

Dear Dr. Goodnow:

I am referring John Jacobs, a 42-year-old man, for a laryngeal examination. I evaluated Mr. Jacobs for a voice disorder on September xx, xxxx. He reported that his voice is "too rough" and that he wanted treatment. He works in noisy construction areas. His history suggests chronic hoarseness and occasional pain in his laryngeal area. My evaluation indicates a harsh and breathy voice with frequent pitch breaks. Mr. Jacobs cannot sustain phonation. His speech intensity drops at the end of his sentences.

I have enclosed a copy of my evaluation report. If there are no contraindications, I plan to start a voice treatment program after your examination. Therefore, please send me a copy of your report. Please call me if you have questions. I thank you for your help.

Yours sincerely,

Sylvia Rodriguez, Ph.D., CCC-SLP
Speech-Language Pathologist

Note to Student Clinicians

Contact your clinic secretary to find out about *thank you* letters written to other professionals. Also, find out about other kinds of letters your clinic sends out.

C.7. PRACTICE IN WRITING
PROFESSIONAL CORRESPONDENCE

C.7.I. A *THANK YOU* LETTER

On the next page, write a *Thank You* letter to a neurologist who has referred to you *an adult patient with aphasia.*

The name of your clinic (L1H)

Date

The name, title, and address of the person receiving the letter.

Describe the client and his or her problem.

Summarize your assessment.

Briefly state your plan for the client (e.g., communication treatment will be offered in twice weekly sessions).

Sign your name.

C.7.I. A *THANK YOU* LETTER

Write your letter. Invent information as needed.

C.7.2. A *REFERRAL* LETTER

On the next page, write A *Referral* letter to a reading specialist to whom you refer a child. Assume that you are treating this child for an oral language disorder and that he or she needs treatment for reading problems.

The name of your clinic (L1H)
Date
The name, title, and address of the person receiving the letter.
Describe the child and his or her problem.
Give a brief history.
Summarize your assessment.
Summarize your treatment targets, procedures, and results.
Request assessment and potential treatment for the child's reading problems.
Sign your name.

C.7.2. A *REFERRAL* LETTER

Write your letter. Invent information as needed.

Note to Student Writers

Please go back and check the entire book to make sure that you have completed all writing assignments. The only method of learning to write well is to write and rewrite. Complete the unfinished assignments and edit the completed ones.

BIBLIOGRAPHY

SOURCES ON CLINICAL REPORT WRITING

The clinical assessment, treatment, and progress reports outlined in this coursebook are based on information presented in the textbooks listed here. If you are not sure of clinical terms, assessment techniques, or treatment procedures, consult the following sources. You also may use textbooks you used in courses on clinical methods, including diagnostic procedures. Ask your supervisor, clinical director, or course instructor to recommend other sources.

Hegde, M. N. (1996). *PocketGuide to assessment in speech-language pathology*. San Diego, CA: Singular Publishing Group.

Hegde, M. N. (1996). *PocketGuide to treatment in speech-language pathology*. San Diego, CA: Singular Publishing Group.

Hegde, M. N. (1998). *Treatment procedures in communicative disorders* (3rd ed.). Austin, TX: Pro-Ed.

Hegde, M. N., & Davis, D. (1995). *Clinical methods and practicum in speech-language pathology* (2nd ed.). San Diego, CA: Singular Publishing Group.

SELECTED BOOKS ON WRITING

Many excellent sources on general, technical, and professional writing are available. Besides the APA *Manual,* students should consult a few of the following books.

American Medical Association. (1989). *American Medical Association manual of style* (8th ed.). Baltimore: Williams & Wilkins.

American Psychological Association. (1994). *Publication manual of the American Psychological Association* (4th ed.). Washington, DC: Author.

Bates, J. D. (1980). *Writing with precision.* Washington, DC: Acropolis Books Ltd.

Burchfield, R. W. (1996). *The new Fowler's modern English usage* (3rd ed.). New York: Oxford University Press.

Follett, W. (1966). *Modern American usage: A guide.* New York: Hill & Wang.

Fowler, H. W. (1987). *A dictionary of modern English usage* (2nd ed., rev.). New York: Oxford University Press.

Hegde, M. N. (1996). *A Singular manual of textbook preparation* (2nd ed.). San Diego, CA: Singular Publishing Group.

International Association of Business Communicators. (1982). *Without bias: A guidebook for non-discriminatory communication* (2nd ed.). New York: Wiley.

Kane, T. (1988). *The new Oxford guide to writing.* New York: Oxford University Press.

Kirszner, L. G., & Mandell, S. R. (1986). *The Holt handbook.* New York: Holt, Rinehart, & Winston.

Li, X., & Crane, M. B. (1993). *Electronic style: A guide to citing electronic information.* Westport, CT: Meckler.

Miller, C., & Swift, K. (1988). *The handbook of nonsexist writing for writers, editors, and speakers* (2nd ed.). New York: Harper & Row.

Modern Language Association. (1988). *MLA handbook for writers of research papers, theses, and dissertations.* New York: Author.

Moore, R. B. (1976). *Racism in the English language.* New York: Council on Interracial Books for Children/Racism and Sexism Resource Center for Educators.

Morris, W., & Morris, M. (1974). *Harper dictionary of contemporary usage.* New York: Harper.

Newman, E. (1975). *A civil tongue.* New York: Warner Books.

Strunk, W., Jr., & White, E. B. (1979). *The elements of style* (3rd ed.). New York: Macmillan.

University of Chicago Press. (1987). *Chicago guide to preparing electronic manuscripts for authors and publishers.* Chicago: Author.

University of Chicago Press. (1993). *The Chicago manual of style* (14th ed., rev.). Chicago: Author.

Zinser, W. (1980). *On writing well: An informal guide to writing nonfiction.* (2nd ed.). New York: Harper & Row.

GLOSSARY

In writing your scientific and professional writing, use the terms as defined in this glossary or *as defined by your instructor or clinical supervisor*. Also, consult books on clinical methods. See the bibliography for a few sources and ask your clinical supervisor for additional sources.

Abstract—A brief summary of a research paper manuscript printed on a separate page (page 2); in the published articles, the abstract is printed on the title page, below the authors and their affiliation.

Ampersand—The character & used in place of *and*; used in reference lists to connect names; not used in regular text except for inside parentheses for multiple author references.

Appendixes—Materials placed at the end of a paper or a chapter to give additional details on selected aspects of what is written in the body of a paper; the preferred plural spelling is *appendixes*, not *appendices*.

Arabic Numerals—The widely used numbering system (e.g., 0, 1 through 10) in many parts of the world including most countries in Europe and the United States; also known as the Hindu-Arabic numerals because of its origin in India; contrasted with roman numerals; the terms *arabic* and *roman* when used to refer to number systems, are not capitalized except when they start a sentence.

Assessment—Clinical procedures designed to diagnose a disorder or evaluate a client's existing and nonexisting communicative behaviors, communicative problems, and potential factors associated with these problems.

Baselines—Measures of communicative or other behaviors before the treatment is started; they help evaluate the client's improvement in treatment; they may be taken on evoked and modeled trials or in conversational speech. *Baselines* and *baserates* can both be nouns; but only baserate can be used as a verb (*baserated*, not *baselined*). Baselines of various communicative behaviors may be established by either using discrete trials or by taking conversational speech and language samples. See **Discrete Baseline Trial**.

Bibliography—A list of all relevant publications on a given topic or field of research; much more comprehensive than a reference list; not attached to a paper or a chapter; may be free-standing; the format may be the same as that of a reference list.

Block Quotation—A quotation of 40 or more words reproduced verbatim from another source, including the author's own words published elsewhere; does not contain quotation marks and is set as a separate paragraph with a rigidly specified format.

Booster Treatment—Treatment given any time after the client was dismissed from the original treatment to maintain clinically established skills; given after a follow-up assessment indicates a need for additional treatment.

CD-ROM—Compact Disk Read-Only Memory; a compact disk that stores a vast amount of information including graphics and sound.

Cliches—Popular, overused, and dull expressions.

Conditioned Generalized Reinforcers—Tokens, money, and such other reinforcers that are effective in a wide range of conditions.

Conditioned Reinforcers—Events that reinforce behaviors because of past learning experiences. The same as *secondary reinforcers.*

Continuous Reinforcement—A schedule in which the clinician reinforces all correct responses.

Conversational Turn Taking—Switching from the role of a speaker to that of a listener and vice versa; a conversational skill taught to persons with language disorders.

Corrective Feedback—Consequences that decrease behaviors; for example, saying "No," "Not correct," "Wrong," and so forth when a client's response is unacceptable.

Criteria—Rules to make various clinical judgments including when to model, when to stop modeling, and when a behavior is trained (e.g., the target is the 90% correct production of the regular plural *s* in words).

Diagnostic Report—A report on the methods and results of an assessment done on a client with a disorder or disease; description of diagnostic procedures and their results; also known as an assessment report.

Discrete Baseline Trial—An opportunity to produce a target response when no reinforcers or corrective feedback is given; may be modeled or evoked; steps are the same as those described under **Discrete Training Trial, Evoked** and **Discrete Training Trial, Modeled** except that no reinforcement or corrective feedback is provided specifically for the correct or incorrect responses; the client may be periodically reinforced for being cooperative and responsive.

Discrete Training Trial, Evoked—An opportunity to produce a target response when the clinician does not model that response; in administering an evoked trial, the clinician:

1. Places the stimulus item in front of the client, or demonstrates the action or event with the help of objects.
2. Asks the predetermined question.
3. Waits a few seconds for the client to respond.
4. If the client's response is correct, reinforces it immediately by verbal praise and any other potential reinforcer.
5. If the client's response is incorrect, immediately gives corrective feedback.
6. Records the response on the recording sheet.
7. Pulls the stimulus item toward herself, or removes it from the client's view.
8. Waits a few seconds to mark the end of the trial.
9. Initiates the next trial.

Discrete Training Trial, Modeled—An opportunity to produce a target response when the clinician models that response; in administering a modeled trial, the clinician:

1. Places the stimulus item in front of the client, or demonstrates the action or event with the help of objects.
2. Asks the predetermined question.
3. Immediately models the correct response.
4. Waits a few seconds for the client to respond.
5. If the client's response is correct, reinforces it immediately by verbal praise and any other potential reinforcer.
6. If the client's response is incorrect, immediately gives corrective feedback.
7. Records the response on the recording sheet.
8. Pulls the stimulus item toward herself, or removes it from the client's view.
9. Waits a few seconds to mark the end of the trial.
10. Initiates the next trial.

E-mail—Electronic mail; sending messages electronically, via a network of computers.

Euphemism—Hiding negative meanings by positive sounding words. For example, the term *residentially challenged* is a positive-sounding term for the *homeless*.

Evoked Trial—A structured opportunity to produce a response when the clinician does not model; presenting a picture and asking a question (e.g., "What is this?") is an example of a discrete trial.

Exemplar—A response that illustrates a target behavior (e.g., *these are two cups* is an exemplar of the regular plural *s*).

Fading—A method of reducing the controlling power of a stimulus while still maintaining the response.

Fixed Interval Schedule—An intermittent schedule of reinforcement in which a response produced after a fixed duration is reinforced.

Fixed Ratio Schedule—An intermittent schedule of reinforcement in which a certain number of responses are required to earn a reinforcer.

Flush-left—Typing the first character flush with the left margin, with no indentation.

Follow-up—Probe or assessment of response maintenance after dismissal from treatment; usually involves taking a new speech and language sample to assess the production of previously taught responses or skills.

Footers—A feature of computer word processors; a full or abbreviated title of a paper or a chapter printed at the bottom of a page; may contain such other information as the chapter number, time and date of printing, and the author name; may be flush-left, centered, or right-aligned; not used in the APA style.

FTP—File Transfer Protocol; electronic means of transferring data from one computer to another via a network of computers.

Functional Outcome—Generalized, broader, and socially and personally meaningful effects of treatment; an overall improvement in communication between clients, their families, and their caregivers.

Generalized Production of Target Responses—Production of responses when the treatment procedure is not in effect; for example, the clinician may take a speech sample without implementing any treatment procedures to see if a child, who has been taught various language structures, uses them; this procedure of assessing generalized production is called probes.

Headings—Subtitles within a paper or a chapter that suggests the subtopic that follows; classified into levels (e.g., level 1 and level 2 headings); not to be confused with a title, headers, page headers (of a manuscript), or running heads.

Headers—A feature of computer word processors; an abbreviated or full title of a paper or a chapter printed on top of each page of a manuscript; may contain additional information including the author's name and time and date of printing; depending on the style used, may be flush-left, centered, or right-aligned; in the APA style, abbreviated and typed right-aligned; contrasted with footers.

IEPs—Individual Educational Plans for children with disabilities or special needs; typically written in educational settings; similar to target behaviors and treatment procedures specified in clinical settings.

IFSPs—Individualized Family Service Plans developed for infants and toddlers and their family members; typically written in educational settings.

Imitation—Learning in which responses take the same form as their stimuli; modeling provides the stimuli; often necessary in the initial stages of treatment.

Informant—A person who gives case history and related information to the clinician; it may be the client himself or herself or another person (e.g., a family member).

Intermediate Response—Responses other than the initial and final used in shaping.

Internet—A high-speed network of computers linked to transfer data from one computer to another; computers may be liked locally, nationally, and internationally; they share standard communication protocols.

Initial Response—The first, simplified component of a target response used in shaping.

Instructions—Verbal stimuli that gain control over other persons' actions; description of how to perform certain actions; often given before modeling a skill for the client.

Intermittent Reinforcement—Reinforcing only some responses or responses produced with some delay between reinforcers.

Intermixed Probes— Procedures of assessing generalized production by alternating trained and untrained stimulus items; typically administered on discrete trials; one trial involves a previously trained stimulus (e.g., the picture of *two cups*, used in training the plural *s*), and the next trial involves an untrained (novel) stimulus (e.g., the picture of *two books*, not used in training); correct responses given to untrained stimuli are counted to calculate the percentage correct probe response rate. See also, **Probes**.

Maintenance strategy—Extension of treatment to natural settings; a collection of methods to help maintain clinically established skills over time; includes such procedures as teaching the client to self-monitor his or her behaviors and training the significant others to prompt and reinforce those behaviors in natural settings.

Manual Guidance—Physical guidance provided to shape a response; gently guiding a child's tongue tip toward the alveolar ridge with a tongue depressor to help the child produce a speech sound is an example of manual guidance; taking the client's hand and pointing to a correct picture is another example.

Mean Length of Utterance (MLU)—A measure of language development; measured as the number of morphemes or words in each utterance and averaged across a collection of utterances.

Modeled Trial— An opportunity to imitate a response when the clinician models it; see **Discrete Trial, Modeled**.

Modeling—The clinician's production of the target response the client is expected to learn; used to teach imitation. (e.g., the clinican might show a picture of a boy running, ask, "What is the boy doing?" and immediately model the response by saying, "Say the boy is running.")

Mood—In grammar, mood refers to various verb forms that indicate whether implied or expressed actions are more or less likely; indicative mood expresses factual statements; subjunctive mood suggests uncertainty; and imperative mood suggests a command or request.

Online—A format of storing information that can be retrieved in an interactive manner; many journals now are online, meaning that they can be searched through the Internet.

Operational Definitions—Scientific definitions that describe how what is defined is measured; clinical treatment targets should be defined operationally (e.g., "I will teach language competence," is not an operational description of a target; "I will teach the following four grammatic morphemes in sentences," followed by a list, is).

Oral-Peripheral Examination—A visual examination of the oral and facial structures to detect gross abnormality; includes several tasks (such as producing certain vowels, moving the tongue, lifting the soft palate) to assess functional integrity of the oral and facial structures; also known as orofacial examination.

Page Header—A brief header printed on each page of a research article (including the title page) except for those containing the figures; consists of two or three words taken from the title of the paper and printed on the upper right-hand corner above or five spaces left of the page number; not to be confused with the running head.

Parallelism—Expressing similar or a series of ideas in similar forms; similar or a series of ideas expressed in different forms violate parallelism, resulting in nonparallel constructions.

Parenthetic Constructions—Phrases within sentences that express ideas that are not integral to those sentences; enclosed within parentheses.

Peer Training—Training peers of clients to evoke and reinforce target behaviors in natural settings; a maintenance strategy.

Positive Reinforcers—Events that, when presented immediately after a response is made, increase the future probability of that response.

Pragmatic Features—Aspects of language use in social contexts; targets of language treatment; include such skills as conversational turn taking and topic maintenance.

Prompts—Special stimuli that increase the probability of a response; prompts may be verbal or nonverbal; similar to hints.

Primary Reinforcers—Unconditioned reinforcers whose effects do not depend upon past learning.

Probe—Procedure to assess generalized production of responses. See also **Intermixed Probes** and **Pure Probes**; discrete trials or conversational speech samples may be used to probe the target behavior production when treatment is not in effect.

Probe Criterion—A rule that says that a trained response is satisfactorily produced without the treatment variables; for example, *95% fluency maintained in conversational speech when the clinician does not reinforce or prompt the target fluency* describes a probe criterion.

Pure probes—Procedures for assessing generalized production with only untrained stimulus items; contrasted with intermixed probes in which trained and untrained stimuli are alternated; for example, in administering pure probes, a clinician may present 20 untrained pictures that show plural objects to assess whether the child will produce the plural *s* with no reinforcement.

Reference List—A list of all and only the works cited in the body of text; follows a prescribed format; always attached to a paper, a chapter, or an entire book; not free-standing; not to be confused with a bibliography.

Reinforcers—Events that follow behaviors and thereby increase the future probability of those behaviors. See also **Positive** and **Negative Reinforcers**.

Right-justification—Printing lines to align with the right margin, as in most printed books; when computer-printed, the words may have uneven spaces between them; not accepted in the APA style.

Running Head—An abbreviated title of a research paper printed flush-left at the top of the title page, but below the page header; printed in all capitals, it does not exceed 50 character spaces including letters, punctuation marks, and spaces between letters.

Schedules of Reinforcement—Different patterns of reinforcement that generate different patterns of responses; includes such schedules as continuous reinforcement (every response is reinforced) and intermittent reinforcement (some responses are not reinforced).

Self-control—A behavior that monitors other behaviors of the same person; a maintenance strategy; clients who are taught to count their errors, for example, have learned to monitor their responses.

Serial Comma—The comma that is used in a series of similar elements including before *and* and *or*, as in *clients, their families, and employers*; *roses, gardenias, or magnolias.*

Shaping—A method of teaching nonexistent responses that are not even imitated. The responses are simplified and taught in an ascending sequence. Also known as *successive approximations.*

Significant Others—People who are important in the lives of clients; includes family members, peers, colleagues, and teachers; training them in prompting and reinforcing a client's target behavior is a maintenance strategy.

Social Reinforcers—A variety of conditioned reinforcers, which include verbal praise.

Subscript—A character or a number printed lower than the rest of the printed line; the lower 1 in X_1 is a subscript.

Superscript—A character or a number printed higher than the rest of the printed line; the elevated D in S^D is a superscript.

Targets—Behaviors a client is taught; communicative skills that are trained.

Telnet—A method of logging on the computers on the Internet; a means of connecting to remote computers.

Terminal Response—The final response targeted in shaping.

Time-out—A period of nonreinforcement imposed response contingently; the typical effect is reduced rate of that response.

Title—The name given to a paper or a chapter; printed on the title page; repeated on every page of a book chapter; printed, in an abbreviated form, on all pages of a research paper; not to be confused with headings in a paper or chapter.

Tokens—Objects that are earned during treatment and exchanged later for back-up reinforcers.

Topic Maintenance—Talking on a single topic for an extended period of time; a language skill taught to persons with language disorders.

Training Criterion—A rule that says that a given target response has been trained; for example, 90% correct responses over a block of trials for a given target response may mean that that response has been trained.

Treatment—In communicative disorders, it is the management of contingent relations between antecedents, responses, and consequences; it is a rearrangement of communicative relationships between a speaker and his or her listener.

Trial—A structured opportunity to produce a response; see **Discrete Training Trial, Evoked** and **Discrete Training Trial, Modeled**.

Variable Interval Schedule—An intermittent reinforcement schedule in which the time duration between reinforcers is varied around an average.

Variable Ratio Schedule—An intermittent reinforcement schedule in which the number of responses needed to earn a reinforcer is varied around an average.

World Wide Web (WWW)—A vast structure of interconnected computers that store electronic files of data that can be retrieved; information is transmitted across the Internet; a graphical environment for creating and storing information.